SOMATIC WORKOUT FOR WEIGHT LOSS

Enhance Flexibility, Strength, and Balance with Low-Impact Exercises for Belly Fat Reduction and Stress Relief

Carlos McDaniel

BONUS INSIDE TO THANK READER FOR PURCHASING THIS BOOK

Inside this book after the conclusion, you will have access to somatic workout tracker journal and the audio version of this book

Table of Contents

Introduction to Somatic Workout for Weight Loss

Clara lived in the center of Evermore, a busy metropolis where life never seemed to calm down. Clara, like many others, juggled the responsibilities of her profession, personal life, and the ongoing fight with her weight. She had tried a variety of training routines, diets, and trends, all promising transformational results. However, nothing appeared to work in the long run. Clara felt estranged from her body, considering it as an opponent rather than an ally in her weight reduction quest.

Clara was browsing through her Facebook feed one day, fatigued and disillusioned after yet another fruitless gym session, when she came across an advertisement for a new guide called "Somatic Workout for Weight Loss." Clara seemed intrigued by the phrase "somatic," which she was unfamiliar with, and determined to learn more. The guide promised more than simply another fitness routine, but rather a journey to reconnect with one's body via conscious movement and awareness.

The tutorial begins with an introduction to somatic exercises, describing how these practices prioritize the internal feeling of movement over the exterior appearance or performance. It claimed to teach readers how to listen to their bodies, detect stress and tension, and employ gentle, conscious movements to relieve and change them.

Clara, skeptical yet interested, purchased the guidebook. As she began to follow its precepts, something inside her began to change. The guide guided her through a series of somatic exercises, beginning with basic breathing techniques and advancing to more sophisticated motions aimed at increasing body awareness and muscle activation. Each chapter included thorough explanations and tales about how these exercises had helped people not just lose weight, but also develop a more harmonious connection with their bodies.

Clara learnt to approach her weight reduction process with love and inquiry, not condemnation and resentment. She realized how distant she had been from her own body, regarding it as a tool to be controlled rather as a partner to be heard. The somatic exercises, with their emphasis on interior experience, helped her to recognize when she was actually hungry, when she was eating out of boredom or stress, and how to appreciate activity for its own purpose, rather than for calorie burn.

After a few months, Clara felt not just lighter in weight but also lighter in spirit. The guide had transformed her body, but also her connection with it. She no longer regarded exercise as a duty, but as a joyful celebration of her body's abilities. Her eating habits spontaneously evolved toward more healthy options, not because she was on a rigorous diet, but because she had learned to listen to her body's true needs.

Clara one day saw an old acquaintance for coffee, who was taken aback by her makeover. Not only did Clara lose weight, but she also exuded a sense of health and pleasure. "What's your secret?" her companion said, hoping to learn about the newest diet fad or strenuous training routine.

Clara grinned, her thoughts returning to the various programs she had attempted before, none of which had taken her to where she was now. "It's not about pushing your body to its limits or following a strict diet," she said. "It's about reconnecting with your body, knowing what it needs, and moving in a way that feels wonderful.

It's about transforming your connection with your body and yourself."

Clara discovered she had unintentionally become an evangelist for the somatic workout guide as she shared her story. She had discovered a long-term way to lose weight and, more significantly, to love herself and accept her physical appearance. The guide had taught her that the key to long-term transformation was to look within and listen to her own body's wisdom, rather than following the current fad or working out the hardest.

Clara's advice to anyone suffering with their weight reduction journey, feeling alienated and dejected, was simple: "Buy the guide." It's more than simply a fitness plan; it's the beginning of a new way of living and being in your body. It's the finest investment you can make in yourself, not just for weight reduction, but also for long-term health and enjoyment."

Overview of Somatic Exercise

Somatic exercise is a type of movement that focuses on internal perception and the experience of the body from inside. This method is based on the idea that the mind and body are inextricably linked, rather than distinct entities. Somatic exercises provide a unique approach to weight loss that goes beyond standard workouts, concentrating on the quality of movement rather than the quantity. This practice promotes a profound awareness of physical sensations, which can lead to more attentive eating habits, lower stress levels, and a better overall lifestyle. By stressing how movements feel rather than how they appear, people are encouraged to move in ways that are therapeutic and nourishing, facilitating weight reduction via a gentle yet profound engagement with the body.

Somatic exercise concepts are strongly aligned with current understandings of neuroplasticity, implying that via attentive movement, people may retrain their neural systems, reduce chronic stress, and enhance metabolism. This retraining process is critical for weight reduction because it tackles the sometimes ignored mental and emotional components of losing extra weight. Somatic practices teach people how to release patterns of holding and tension in their bodies, which can be impediments to optimal metabolism and weight control. This comprehensive approach not only helps to reduce physical weight but also relieves the psychological strain that frequently comes with the weight reduction journey, making the process more sustainable and pleasurable.

Somatic workouts for weight reduction include a range of strategies, including slow, controlled motions that need intense attention and awareness. These exercises frequently begin with the breath, which is utilized to increase physiological awareness and inspire movement from a state of centeredness. As participants become more aware of their internal states, they may engage in activities such as pandiculation, which involves tightening and then gently releasing muscles to teach the body more efficient movement patterns. This muscle re-education can result in improved posture and movement efficiency, which not only helps to burn calories more effectively but also prevents injuries that could hinder weight reduction attempts.

Somatic exercises, unlike high-intensity workouts, do not focus on calorie burning or muscular depletion. Instead, the emphasis is on recalibrating the body's perception of itself, which might result in a natural rebalancing of weight. This approach recognizes that weight increase is frequently an indication of separation from the body, whether due to stress, sedentary lifestyles, or incorrect eating patterns. Somatic exercise promotes a deeper connection with the body, which can lead to healthier lifestyle choices, such as those linked to nutrition and physical activity, and so aids in weight reduction.

Individual demands and situations must be taken into account while designing somatic workouts for weight loss. Unlike one-size-fits-all workout plans, somatic practices may be adjusted to each individual's body's specific needs. This customisation ensures that workouts are both effective and accessible, lowering the risk of injury and boosting the chance of program adherence. This individualized approach respects the body's boundaries and potential, promoting progressive growth that is consistent with the body's natural cycles and ability to adapt.

Another significant advantage of somatic exercise in the context of weight reduction is its potential to lower stress, which is a recognized cause to weight gain and a barrier to weight loss. Individuals can confront the stress-weight link head on by practicing relaxation and chronic tension release techniques. This stress reduction is accomplished not via distraction or detachment, but through a greater sense of body awareness and present. Cortisol levels, a hormone linked to belly fat storage, can fall when stress levels fall, assisting weight loss attempts and improving general health.

Finally, somatic exercise provides a compassionate and complete approach to weight loss, respecting the body's knowledge and the complicated connections between mind, body, and environment. Somatic workouts for weight reduction encourage substantial transformation by moving the attention away from outward markers of success and toward interior feelings of movement and wellness. This transition is about more than just reducing weight; it's about reestablishing a healthy connection with the body, which leads to long-term improvements that go well beyond the physical sphere. Somatic practices take people on a path of self-discovery, teaching them how to manage their weight loss journey with mindfulness, grace, and a deep respect for the body's intrinsic knowledge.

Benefits of Somatic Exercise for Weight Loss

Somatic exercise, an innovative method to weight reduction, emphasizes the internal sensation of movement rather than the exterior results of exercise, resulting in a significant shift in how people participate with their fitness journey. This practice stresses the value of mindfulness and body awareness, urging practitioners to listen to their bodies' signals and demands. Somatic exercise helps people comprehend the core reasons of their eating patterns and physical inactivity by building a stronger connection between mind and body, which frequently leads to better long-term weight loss and health benefits.

The premise of relieving muscular tension and chronic stress, both of which are common hurdles to efficient weight control, is central to somatic exercise theory. Individuals can learn to detect and release stress patterns that relate to emotional eating and sedentary lifestyles via mild, mindful exercises. This release not only promotes physical mobility and pain relief, but it also increases metabolic efficiency, allowing the body to burn calories more effectively and regulate hunger.

Another notable advantage of somatic exercise for weight loss is its ability to reduce stress. High levels of stress are associated with weight gain, particularly in the abdomen area, due to the synthesis of the hormone cortisol. Somatic techniques, which emphasize relaxation and attentive awareness, might help decrease stress levels, potentially lowering cortisol production and weight gain. This calm state also promotes healthier sleep patterns, which help with weight reduction by regulating hormones that affect appetite and fullness.

Unlike standard exercise regimens, which frequently emphasize high intensity and volume as major techniques for weight loss, somatic exercise promotes deliberate, focused motions. This method not only reduces the danger of injury, but also makes exercise more accessible to a wider range of people, independent of fitness level or mobility. Somatic exercise enhances the chance of long-term commitment to a physical activity plan, which is important for weight reduction and health.

Somatic exercise also helps to improve proprioception, or the body's capacity to perceive its location and motions in space. Enhanced proprioception improves coordination and balance, making physical activity safer and more effective. As people become more aware of their bodies, they may adapt their motions to be more effective, decreasing wasted energy and optimizing the benefits of their exercises. This increased bodily awareness enables the identification of personal physical limitations, lowering the danger of overexertion and injury.

Somatic exercise is holistic in nature, which means it not only helps with weight reduction but also promotes to general well-being. Practitioners commonly report enhanced sensations of calm, pleasure, and body satisfaction, which can help to alleviate the negative self-image and mental discomfort that are common with obesity and weight issues. This favorable alteration in self-perception and mental wellness may lessen dependency on food for emotional comfort, aiding weight reduction attempts.

To summarize, somatic exercise is a holistic approach to weight management that goes beyond standard approaches by addressing the physical, emotional, and psychological elements of health. Its advantages go beyond calorie burning to include stress reduction, increased bodily awareness, and a healthy connection with food and exercise. Individuals who incorporate somatic techniques into their weight loss journey might achieve better long-term outcomes, shifting their approach to health and wellbeing from struggle and frustration to harmony and awareness.

How Somatic Workouts Complement Traditional Weight Loss Methods

Somatic exercises provide a distinct approach to weight loss that complements standard approaches by emphasizing the internal sensation of movement and body awareness. Unlike traditional exercise programs, which frequently stress intensity, length, and particular physical objectives, somatic exercises urge people to pay attention to their bodies. This mindfulness-based approach promotes a better awareness of bodily indicators such as hunger and satiety, stress levels, and emotional well-being, all of which play important roles in weight control. Individuals who have a greater sense of body awareness can make more educated decisions regarding diet, exercise, and lifestyle behaviors that aid in weight loss.

Traditional weight management strategies frequently emphasise the necessity of calorie control and regular exercise. While these components are necessary for weight loss, they might occasionally cause a disconnect with the body's natural signals. Somatic workouts bridge this gap by reintegrating the mind and body, educating people to identify and respect their own body's requirements and limitations. This technique can lead to a more lasting and joyful weight reduction journey since people learn to engage in physical activities that they like rather than perceiving exercise as a punishment.

Somatic exercises have stress-reduction effects that supplement typical weight-loss measures. High levels of stress can undermine weight reduction attempts by increasing cravings for unhealthy meals and delaying metabolism. Somatic activities, such as deep breathing and mindful movement, can assist to reduce stress and its detrimental effects on weight. Individuals who include these routines into their daily routine can overcome one of the hidden barriers to weight reduction, making it simpler to stick to good food and activity regimens.

Furthermore, somatic training can enhance physical functions that are necessary for successful weight loss. These routines help the body complete a variety of activities more effectively by emphasizing movements that improve flexibility, balance, and muscular strength. Improved physical function can result in more exercise, higher calorie burns, and, eventually, weight loss. This comprehensive approach guarantees that the body remains strong and competent, lowering the chance of injury and allowing people to live an active lifestyle for the long term.

Another important way somatic workouts supplement standard approaches is in terms of motivation and involvement. Traditional workout routines can become repetitive or stressful, resulting in a loss of enthusiasm. Somatic exercises, which focus on inward experience and personal discovery, are a novel alternative that may reignite interest in physical activity. The novelty and profundity of somatic activities may keep people interested and inquiring about their bodies, encouraging a positive attitude toward fitness and wellbeing.

Somatic workouts also target the psychological components of weight loss, which are sometimes disregarded in standard approaches. These routines, which promote a caring and nonjudgmental attitude toward the body, can help people overcome negative self-talk and body image issues that impede weight reduction. This positive psychological shift is critical for creating a healthy connection with food and exercise, providing the groundwork for long-term improvement. Individuals who learn to respect their bodies and their potential are more inclined to care for themselves and make decisions that benefit their general well-being.

Somatic exercises provide a valuable supplement to standard weight reduction strategies by addressing the complex interaction of mind, body, and emotions in the quest of health and fitness. Individuals who incorporate somatic techniques into their weight reduction approach might have a more balanced, sustained, and enjoyable route to their objectives. This comprehensive approach not only improves physical health but also promotes mental and emotional well-being, making it an effective ally in the search for long-term weight loss and a better lifestyle.

Getting Started

Preparing Your Space for Somatic Exercise

Creating a favorable setting for somatic exercise is critical for people beginning on a weight reduction journey with mindful movement. The environment in which one practices is critical in developing the profound connection between mind and body that somatic exercises seek to attain. As a result, it is critical to create an environment that not only allows for free mobility but also promotes mental quiet and attention. A tranquil and welcoming environment may considerably improve the efficacy of the exercises by reducing distractions and offering a safe refuge for exploration and growth.

The first step in prepping your environment is to provide plenty of room for mobility. Somatic exercises frequently entail fluid motions and stretches that demand a significant amount of space. Clearing a defined space of furniture and debris allows for the physical freedom required for these activities. This wide area represents a dedication to your health and well-being, acting as both a physical and symbolic clearing for personal growth. It is critical that this space allows you to fully extend out in all directions, so that your somatic practice is not hampered by the fear of colliding with things.

Lighting helps to set the tone for somatic activity. Natural light is especially good since it improves one's attitude and energy levels, making a workout session more enjoyable. If natural light isn't available, gentle, warm lighting can help to create a peaceful environment that promotes relaxation and contemplation. The idea is to establish a balance between enough illumination to see clearly and a softness that fosters a sense of serenity and quiet.

Another thing to consider is the room's temperature. Comfort is essential in somatic activity; therefore, the environment should be neither too hot nor too cold. A suitable temperature keeps the body calm and open to the workouts. It keeps the muscles from tensing up, which is necessary for participating in the focused motions associated with somatic training. Before commencing your practice, regulate the temperature of the space to a suitable level using fans, heaters, or open windows.

Incorporating natural or personal features might help to enhance the space's mood. Plants, for example, may enhance air quality while also adding life and vitality to a space. Similarly, personal artifacts that elicit emotions of calm, joy, or inspiration can help to personalize the setting and make the practice more meaningful. These features serve as subtle reminders of the objective of your weight reduction quest, as well as the holistic nature of physical activity.

Sound is another important component in creating an appropriate environment for somatic activities. Some people prefer silence, relying on the natural noises of their movements and breath to help them focus inside. Others may find that calm, rhythmic music or natural sounds aid in achieving a meditative state, strengthening the mind-body connection. Experimenting with diverse aural settings will help you figure out what works best for your somatic practice, making it a more successful tool for weight reduction and self-discovery.

Finally, privacy is essential in a somatic exercise setting. The practice frequently includes profound personal introspection and vulnerability; thus, it is critical to feel safe from interruptions or inquisitive eyes. Whether it's a room with a closed door, an isolated nook of a bigger area, or a private location in nature, guaranteeing seclusion promotes the openness and receptivity required for somatic practice. It enables for a more profound connection with the exercises, devoid of self-consciousness and external evaluation, making each session a genuine retreat inside oneself.

Preparing your area for somatic exercise entails building a sanctuary for development, healing, and transformation, in addition to the physical environment. This preparation is an important step on the route to weight loss and well-being, laying the groundwork for a practice that benefits not only the body but also the mind and soul.

Equipment and Materials Needed

A somatic workout for weight reduction involves little equipment, demonstrating the practice's emphasis on internal experience and bodily awareness over external instruments. However, a few properly chosen objects may improve the exercise, making it more efficient and pleasurable. The first item of necessary equipment is a comfortable, non-slip yoga mat. This creates a sturdy surface for a wide range of workouts and activities, assuring safety and comfort. A good mat supports the body during floor exercises and eliminates the possibility of slipping, which is especially crucial when doing focused, controlled movements that emphasize alignment and balance.

Another important component is comfortable, breathable gear that provides a complete range of motion. Unlike traditional workouts, which may require specific types of athletic wear, somatic exercises necessitate clothing that does not restrict movement or distract from the internal sensations of the exercise. Clothing should be viewed as a tool for connecting with the body, rather than a fashion statement or performance booster. The appropriate attire will allow participants to move freely, increasing the effectiveness of the exercises and overall experience.

A number of props might help people who want to improve their somatic practice. Foam rollers and massage balls are ideal tools for self-myofascial release, since they assist to relieve muscular tension and promote blood circulation. These instruments are especially effective for warming up the body before more intense activities and cooling down afterwards, which aids in recovery and prevents damage. They also help to develop deeper body awareness by identifying points of tension and learning how to relax them consciously.

Resistance bands are another flexible item that may be used with somatic activities. They may be used to provide light resistance to activities, allowing you to improve strength without using large weights. Resistance bands are especially useful for targeting smaller muscle groups and improving proprioception (the body's ability to perceive its own position in space). By incorporating these bands into somatic exercises, people can improve muscle tone and endurance while remaining true to the principles of mindful movement.

A stability ball can also be an effective addition to somatic workouts, engaging core muscles and improving balance. Exercises performed on a stability ball test the body's equilibrium, necessitating a high level of body awareness to maintain balance. This not only strengthens the core, but also improves coordination and posture, all of which are necessary for efficient movement and weight loss. The ball can be used for a variety of exercises, ranging from basic seated movements to more difficult balance and strength exercises.

A journal can be an effective tool for those who want to keep track of their progress and stay connected to their practice even when they are not on the mat. Recording experiences, sensations, challenges, and achievements sheds light on the personal journey of reconnecting with one's body through somatic practice. It can also be used as a motivational tool, reminding people of their progress and what they've learned about their bodies and themselves.

Finally, making a welcoming and comfortable practice environment is essential. This could include having enough space to move freely, some calming decor or plants, and a speaker for playing gentle music or leading somatic exercise sessions. The environment should promote relaxation and focus, allowing practitioners to forget about the day's stresses and fully engage with their somatic workout. While the equipment and materials required for somatic workouts are minimal, each contributes to a deeper connection with the body, improving the overall experience and effectiveness of the practice for weight loss and well-being.

Understanding Your Body's Signals

Understanding your body's cues is an important part of incorporating somatic workouts into your weight reduction quest. This technique goes beyond typical fitness measurements like calories burnt or miles ran to explore the subtle dialog between mind and body. The first step in this discourse is to understand the distinction between bodily and emotional hunger. Physical hunger develops gradually and may be filled with a range of foods, however emotional hunger appears unexpectedly and requires specialized comfort foods. Somatic exercises promote this awareness by encouraging a conscious connection to body sensations, allowing people to respond to their genuine nutritional needs rather than eating in response to their emotions.

Somatic workouts can teach people how to recognize tension and relaxation levels in their bodies. Physical indicators of stress include clenched muscles, shallow breathing, and an increased heart rate. Individuals who become attentive to these signals can use somatic strategies to actively lower stress levels, which is important because elevated stress can contribute to overeating and weight gain. Deep diaphragmatic breathing, mild stretching, and mindful movement can help with weight control by shifting the body from a stressed to a relaxed state, reducing stress-induced eating patterns.

Fatigue is another important indication to recognize. In today's fast-paced world, it's normal to use coffee or sugar to get through the day, neglecting the body's need for slumber. Somatic workouts encourage the perception of exhaustion as an indication that the body requires rest. Listening to this signal can help you avoid overtraining, lower your chance of injury, and maintain a balanced approach to fitness. Adequate rest is vital for weight reduction because it promotes muscle regeneration, hormone balance, and general health.

Hydration cues are equally significant. Frequently, the body's thirst signal is misunderstood for hunger, resulting in needless eating. Somatic practice promotes acute awareness of the body's fluid requirements, differentiating between thirst and hunger. This awareness promotes weight reduction by ensuring that people drink enough water, keep hydrated, and avoid eating additional calories when they truly need fluids.

Somatic workouts also improve proprioception, or the ability to perceive one's own body's location in space. This awareness is essential for executing workouts properly and securely. Individuals with improved proprioception can prevent injury and activate muscles more efficiently during workouts, resulting in higher weight reduction results. This internal awareness of movement and alignment assists in doing exercises with accuracy, enhancing their benefits and efficiency.

Understanding the signals of the body also includes emotional awareness. Emotions have a significant impact on physical health, influencing eating habits and motivation to exercise. Somatic workouts help people connect with their emotions by noticing how sensations like sorrow, love, and worry appear in the body. This emotional literacy can help people make better choices by encouraging them to eat for food rather than as an emotional response, and to enjoy exercising rather than seeing it as a punishment.

Finally, responding to your body's messages promotes a strong sense of self-compassion and acceptance. This mentality is essential for long-term weight loss. Rather of penalizing the body for perceived shortcomings, somatic exercises instill the importance of appreciation for the body's strengths and resiliency. This good relationship with the body encourages continued care and respect, which influences not just exercise and eating habits but also general quality of life. Individuals who practice somatics learn not just to read but also to heed their bodies' messages, laying the groundwork for long-term health and weight loss.

Setting Realistic Goals

Setting realistic objectives is essential for success in any weight reduction journey, especially when including somatic workouts into the routine. This method encourages individuals to integrate their goals with the complex awareness of their bodies that somatic activities foster. Recognizing the significance of this alignment entails realizing that weight reduction is about more than just losing pounds; it is also about developing a deeper connection with the body. It entails setting objectives that are not just based on the scale, but also on increasing physiological awareness, flexibility, strength, and general well-being.

When beginning a somatic workout program for weight loss, It is critical to establish goals that mirror the principles of somatic exercise: mindfulness, bodily awareness, and stress reduction. This might include attempting to become more aware of the body's hunger and fullness signals, avoiding emotional eating, or improving posture and activity habits. Such objectives help with weight reduction indirectly by addressing the habits and behaviors that lead to weight gain. They provide a broader perspective on health and fitness, stressing the value of exercise technique above quantity.

Realistic goal setting in the context of somatic training entails accepting the body's existing state and limitations. Instead of striving for quick weight reduction, which can lead to dissatisfaction and injury, objectives should be set to increase strength, flexibility, and body composition over time. This method guarantees that the body can safely adjust to increased levels of activity and stress, lowering the danger of burnout or disillusionment. Understanding that improvement in somatic techniques generally manifests as subtle alterations in body awareness and movement efficiency rather than dramatic changes on the scale might aid in setting realistic expectations.

Setting realistic objectives requires taking into account the time and resources available for practice. Somatic workouts need a level of attention and contemplation that may not be feasible with a hectic schedule. Setting objectives that take into account these practical limits ensures that the commitment to somatic exercise remains sustained. It may include beginning with shorter, more regular sessions to establish a practice habit, then progressively increasing the duration and intensity as time permits and the body grows acclimated to the exercises.

Another important feature of somatic fitness programs is to include feedback and reflection in goal setting. Regularly monitoring progress toward goals enables modifications depending on what is and isn't working. This introspective practice aligns with the somatic emphasis on interior experience and physical feedback-driven modification. It promotes a dynamic approach to goal planning, in which objectives shift as people gain a better awareness of their bodies and needs.

Goals for somatic workouts and weight loss should include self-compassion and patience. Weight reduction is a journey with unavoidable ups and downs, and somatic techniques can help people navigate it more easily and with less self-criticism. Setting objectives that recognize the importance of self-care and the non-linear nature of weight reduction helps promote resilience and a healthier body image. This attitude helps to alleviate the disappointment that might follow setbacks by viewing them as chances for learning and progress.

Finally, setting realistic objectives in a somatic fitness program for weight reduction is about achieving balance in mind, body, and spirit. It is about creating goals that respect the body's wisdom, gently push its boundaries, and appreciate its abilities. Such aims not only set the way for long-term weight loss, but also for a deeper, more sensitive sense of being in one's body. This all-encompassing approach to goal planning guarantees that the path to weight reduction is just as satisfying as the destination, instilling a lifetime dedication to health and wellness.

Foundational Somatic Exercises

Breathing Techniques for Weight Loss

Breathing methods are essential in somatic workouts, acting as basic exercises that can considerably improve the weight reduction process. These approaches not only increase oxygenation and metabolic processes, but they also promote a stronger connection between mind and body, which is essential for long-term weight loss. Individuals who focus on their breath can engage their parasympathetic nervous system, lowering stress and thereby alleviating one of the underlying causes of weight gain: stress-induced eating and hormone imbalances.

Diaphragmatic Breathing

This is a fundamental somatic activity that promotes complete oxygen exchange and activates the body's relaxation reactions.

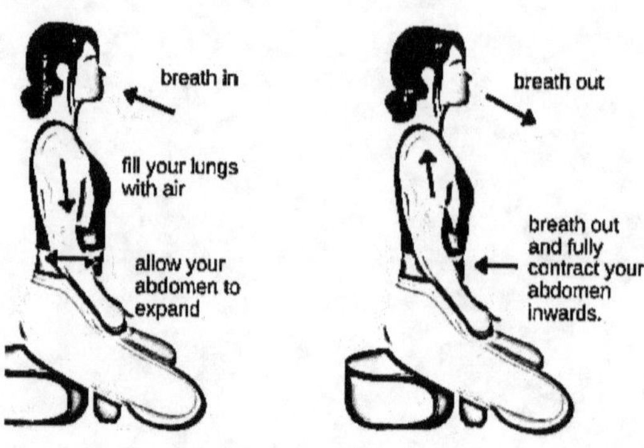

Instructions:

- ✓ Lie on your back with knees bent and feet flat on the floor. Place one hand on your chest and another on your abdomen.

- ✓ Inhale slowly via your nose, ensuring that your diaphragm (not your chest) inflates with enough air to cause a stretch in your lungs.

- ✓ Pause slightly at the peak of each inhalation, then gently exhale through your mouth, using your abdominal muscles to force out all of the air.

- ✓ Repeat this exercise for 5-10 minutes every day, concentrating on the rise and fall of your belly rather than your chest.

Benefits: Diaphragmatic breathing improves oxygenation, detoxification, and relaxation, lowering the risk of stress eating. It also increases core muscular stability, which is good for posture and athletic performance.

Rhythmic Breathing

Rhythmic breathing integrates breath and movement and can be used during somatic exercises or any physical activity to improve endurance and efficiency.

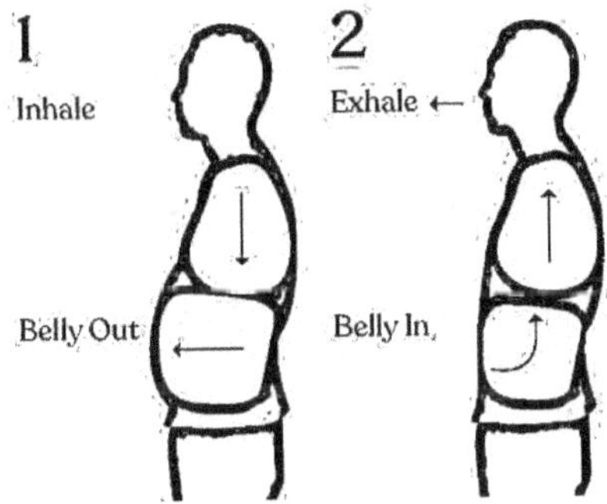

Instructions:

- ✓ Start in a comfortable sitting or standing position.
- ✓ Start with a steady, natural breath cycle, then begin to coordinate your motions with your breath. For example, when inhaling, extend or stretch your arms, and when exhaling, fold or shrink them.

✓ For many minutes, continue to engage in soft, flowing motions that correspond to the rhythm of your breath, with the goal of creating a harmonic balance between movement and breath.

Benefits: This strategy boosts cardiovascular efficiency, lowers tiredness, and heightens the relaxing benefits of exercise on the mind and body, promoting a healthier approach to weight reduction.

4-7-8 Breath

This approach, known for its capacity to produce calm and reduce tension, is especially beneficial for regulating food cravings and emotional eating.

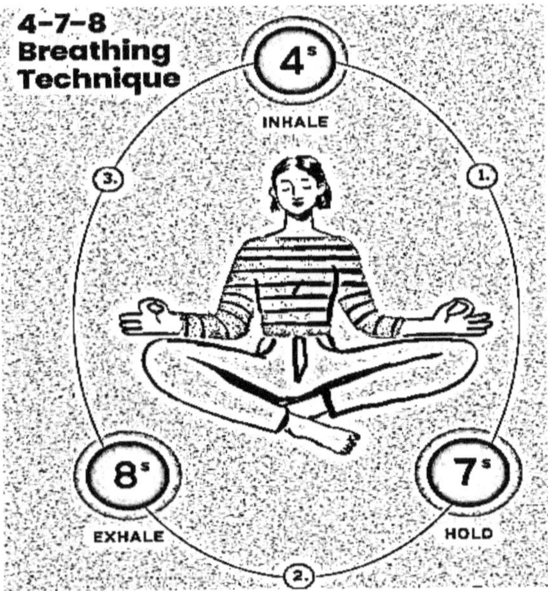

Instructions:

- Sit with your back straight or lie down in a comfortable posture.

- Close your mouth and take a calm breath through your nose for a mental count of four.

- Hold your breath for seven counts.

- Exhale completely through your lips, generating a whoosh sound to the count of eight.

- This completes a single cycle. Repeat the pattern three more times, totaling four breaths.

Benefits: The 4-7-8 breathing method regulates the stress response, which can aid with weight reduction by reducing stress-related eating and enhancing sleep quality.

Incorporating these breathing methods into a somatic workout for weight reduction provides a more comprehensive approach to health and wellness. They not only provide physical advantages, such as increased metabolic rate and workout performance, but they also promote mental and emotional equilibrium. This balanced approach can help people build a more aware connection with their body and food, promoting weight reduction and general health. Regularly doing these breathing exercises can result in considerable gains in stress management, respiratory efficiency, and body awareness—all of which are essential components of a successful weight reduction journey.

Basic Somatic Movements to Enhance Body Awareness

Somatic exercises, a crucial component of somatic workouts, are intended to increase body awareness, which is essential for weight reduction and overall well-being. These motions emphasize the interior sense of movement, fostering a conscious connection between the mind and body. Individuals with increased body awareness can better comprehend their bodily demands, handle stress, and adopt healthier lifestyle patterns. Here, we'll look at some fundamental somatic motions, how to do them, and the benefits they provide in terms of weight reduction.

Pandiculation

- ✓ Begin by resting on your back, noticing your breath and how your body feels against the earth.
- ✓ Slowly stretch your arms aloft and point your toes, expanding your body as much as is comfortable, similar to a morning stretch. Hold this stretch and take a big breath in.

✓ As you exhale, let go of the stretch and allow your body to relax. Observe the sense of release and how different sections of your body feel.

✓ Repeat this technique 3-5 times, concentrating on different parts of the body that may be tense or tight.

Benefits: Pandiculation resets muscle length and lowers muscular tension, increasing flexibility and lowering the risk of injury. It also promotes mindfulness and body awareness, which aids in stress reduction and is essential for controlling cortisol levels, which can impact weight.

The Cat-Cow Stretch

To perform the Cat-Cow Stretch, position yourself on your hands and knees with your wrists under your shoulders and knees under your hips.

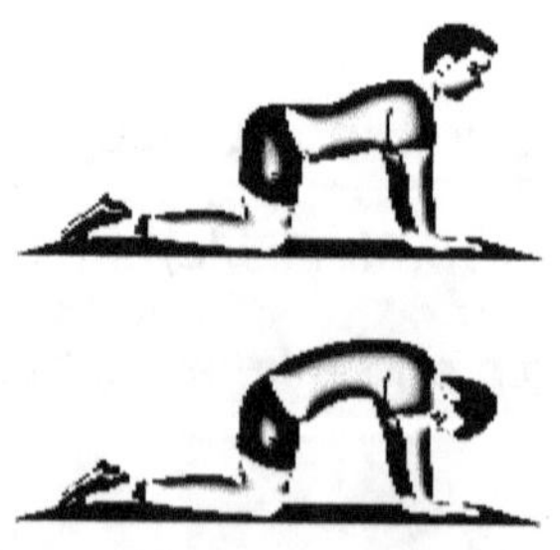

- ✓ Inhale while slowly arching your back downwards and elevating your head and tailbone to the sky (Cow pose).
- ✓ Exhale while rounding your back upwards, tucking your chin to your chest and pulling your navel closer your spine (Cat pose).
- ✓ Continue to alternate gently between these two postures for 5-10 cycles, concentrating on the sense of movement in your spine.

Benefits: This exercise increases spinal flexibility and helps relieve stress in the back and neck. It promotes deeper breathing, which increases oxygen flow and assists in relaxation and stress reduction, hence maintaining a healthy metabolism.

The Pelvic Tilt

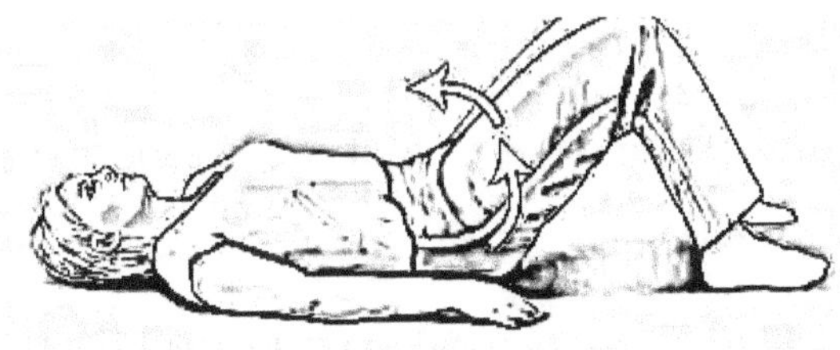

- ✓ Lie on your back, knees bent, feet flat on the floor, arms by your sides.

- ✓ Inhale to prepare your body, then exhale while gently tilting your pelvis towards your ribs and flattening your lower back into the floor.
- ✓ Inhale gently and return to the beginning posture, allowing your lower back to bend naturally.
- ✓ Perform 10-15 repetitions, paying particular attention to pelvic movement and core muscular activation.

Benefits: Pelvic tilts develop abdominal muscles and enhance lower back stability, resulting in a stronger core. A strong core is necessary for appropriate posture, efficient movement, and injury avoidance, all of which promote an active lifestyle and weight reduction.

Hamstring Stretch with Somatic Awareness

- ✓ Lie on your back with one knee bent, foot on the floor, and other leg stretched straight up to the ceiling.
- ✓ Using both hands, gently pull the rear of the thigh of the extended leg towards you while maintaining the leg as straight as possible.

- ✓ Rather of holding the stretch in place, slowly release and re-engage it, going in and out of it with each breath.
- ✓ After 3-5 cycles, swap legs and repeat, paying attention to the feelings in your hamstrings and throughout your body.

Benefits: This dynamic method of stretching the hamstrings enhances flexibility without activating the muscle's stretch reflex, resulting in deeper and more effective lengthening. Improved hamstring flexibility can improve movement efficiency while also lowering the risk of lower back discomfort, making physical activity more accessible and pleasurable.

Integrating these fundamental somatic movements into a weight reduction program increases body awareness, resulting in more mindful eating, improved stress management, and a stronger connection to the body's hunger and fullness signals. Furthermore, the enhanced flexibility, strength, and stability obtained from these workouts promotes a more active lifestyle, enabling long-term weight loss. Somatic activities foster a positive body image and a compassionate approach to weight management, promoting long-term health and well-being.

Aligning Body and Mind for Optimal Performance

Aligning the body and mind is a fundamental aspect of enhancing weight loss efforts, especially when integrating somatic workouts into your routine. Somatic exercises, by their very nature, are designed to foster a deep, intuitive connection between physical movements and mental awareness, creating a holistic approach to health and fitness. This harmonious alignment is crucial for achieving optimal performance in any workout regimen, as it ensures that every exercise is performed with full consciousness and intent, maximizing its benefits.

To begin aligning body and mind, start with focused breathing exercises. This can be as simple as sitting or lying in a comfortable position and paying attention to your breath. Try to:

✓ Inhale deeply through the nose, allowing your abdomen to expand, then exhale slowly through the mouth. This type of breathing helps to calm the mind and prepare the body for physical activity.

✓ Engage in a mindful body scan. From your seated or lying position, mentally scan your body from head to toe, noting any areas of tension or discomfort. This practice encourages mental awareness of the physical state, promoting a closer connection to bodily sensations.

Incorporate gentle stretching into your routine to further this alignment. Stretching with mindfulness means:

✓ Paying attention to the sensations in your muscles and joints as you gently stretch each part of your body. Acknowledge how each stretch feels, and breathe into any areas of tightness, using your breath to facilitate a deeper release.

✓ Practicing dynamic stretches that involve movement, such as arm circles or hip rotations, can also help in syncing movement with breath, enhancing body awareness.

Visualization techniques are a powerful tool for aligning body and mind. Before starting your workout, visualize:

✓ Completing your exercises with ease and strength. Imagine your muscles working in perfect harmony, and picture yourself achieving your weight loss goals. This mental rehearsal can enhance motivation and focus during your workout.

The practice of grounding is essential in somatic workouts. Grounding exercises, such as standing barefoot and imagining roots growing from your feet into the ground, can:

Help center your mind, reduce anxiety, and increase your presence in the now, making your workout more effective and enjoyable.

Somatic movements, like the pelvic tilt or cat-cow stretch, are designed to improve flexibility and core strength while also enhancing mental focus. To perform these exercises:

- ✓ Focus on the slow, controlled movement of your body, paying attention to the alignment of your spine and the engagement of your core muscles. This not only improves physical strength but also encourages a meditative state of mind.

The benefits of aligning body and mind through somatic exercises are manifold. Firstly, this alignment enhances the efficiency of your workouts, as a focused mind can better direct energy to the muscles being worked, leading to more effective fat burning and muscle building. Secondly, it increases body awareness, helping to prevent injury by ensuring that exercises are performed correctly. Thirdly, the stress reduction achieved through mindful exercises can decrease cortisol levels, a hormone that can contribute to weight gain, especially around the midsection.

Furthermore, the practice of somatic exercises with an aligned mind and body can lead to improved sleep patterns and overall well-being, both of which are essential for weight loss and maintenance. By integrating these practices into your weight loss journey, you not only work towards a healthier body but also cultivate a more peaceful, present mind, enhancing your overall quality of life.

Somatic Warm-Up Routines

Gentle Stretches to Prepare Your Body

Gentle stretches are an essential component of somatic warm-up regimens, especially those geared toward weight reduction goals. These stretches are intended to awaken the body, increase body awareness, and prepare the muscles and joints for the more energetic exercises that will follow. Unlike standard static stretches, somatic stretching emphasizes the quality of movement and the mental sensation of stretching, fostering a strong bond between the mind and body. This attentive approach can considerably help with weight reduction by increasing flexibility, lowering the chance of injury, and making the body more sensitive to exercise.

Neck Release Stretch

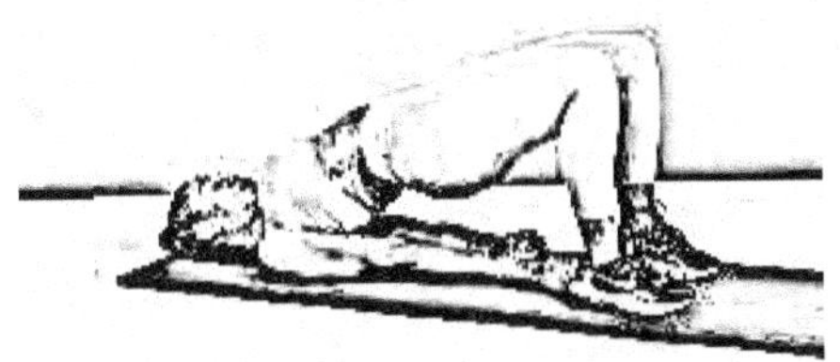

- ✓ Start in a comfortable sitting or standing position, with your spine extended.
- ✓ Gently drop your right ear to your right shoulder while maintaining your left shoulder relaxed and away from your ear.
- ✓ Hold for a second until you feel a stretch on the left side of your neck.
- ✓ Roll your chin slowly towards your chest, then towards your left shoulder, in a semi-circular motion.
- ✓ Repeat this moderate rolling motion 2-3 times before rotating to the opposite side.

Benefits: Reduces strain in the neck and upper shoulders, where stress can gather and affect posture and breathing habits.

Cat-Cow Stretch

- ✓ Begin on your hands and knees in a tabletop posture, placing your wrists under your shoulders and knees under your hips.
- ✓ Inhale as you arch your back, tilt your pelvis up, and raise your head and tailbone to the ceiling (Cow pose).
- ✓ Exhale while rounding your back, lowering your chin to your chest and pulling your navel toward your spine (Cat pose).
- ✓ Continue this movement for 5-10 cycles, following your breath.

Benefits: Improves spinal flexibility and awareness, promotes deeper breathing, and warms up core muscles to maintain posture.

Side Stretch

- ✓ Stand with your feet hip-width apart or sit tall on a chair.
- ✓ Raise your arms upward, interlacing your fingers and maintaining your palms facing up.
- ✓ Gently lean to the right, keeping both feet firmly on the ground or both sit bones on the chair, and feel a stretch on your left side.

✓ Hold for a few breaths before returning to the middle and repeating on the opposite side.

Benefits: Opens up the side body, increasing lung capacity and promotes good alignment, which is essential for efficient breathing and movement.

Pelvic Tilts

✓ Lie on your back, knees bent, feet flat on the floor, hip-width apart.

✓ Inhale to prepare your body, then exhale, gently tilting your pelvis towards your face and flattening your lower back into the floor.

✓ Inhale, return to the beginning posture, and tilt your pelvis away from you, arching your lower back slightly.

✓ Repeat this action gently for 5-10 times.

Benefits: Engages and warms the core muscles, increases pelvic mobility, and heightens awareness of spinal alignment.

Leg Swings

- ✓ Stand alongside a wall or strong chair for support and balance.
- ✓ Swing one leg forth and back in a smooth manner while maintaining your body erect and engaged.
- ✓ Swing 10-15 times with one leg before switching to the other.

Benefits: Stretches the hips and hamstrings, prepares the legs for weight-bearing movements, and enhances dynamic balance and coordination.

Arm Circles

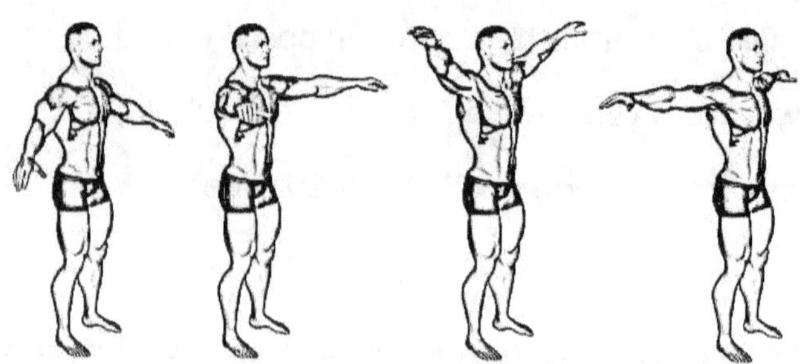

- ✓ Stand with feet shoulder-width apart and arms outstretched to the sides at shoulder height.
- ✓ Slowly spin your arms in small circles, gradually increasing the size of each circle.
- ✓ After 10-15 seconds, reverse the directions of the circles.

Benefits: Warms up the shoulder joints, increases blood flow to the arms, and improves upper body mobility, which is required for full-body somatic exercises.

Incorporating these mild stretches into your warm-up routines has several benefits, especially in terms of weight loss. They not only prepare the body physiologically by boosting blood flow, improving flexibility, and lowering the chance of injury, but they also prime the mind by encouraging mindfulness and body awareness. This comprehensive preparation is required for effective somatic exercises, as it increases the body's receptivity to exercise and supports long-term weight loss. By beginning each training session with these mild stretches, people may assure a safer, more pleasurable, and successful exercise experience.

Dynamic Movement to Increase Heart Rate

Dynamic movement is essential in somatic warm-up programs, especially those geared toward weight loss. These motions are intended to gently prepare the body for exercise by raising heart rate, boosting blood flow, and improving range of motion, all while emphasizing physiological awareness and mindfulness. Individuals may establish a smooth transition between a state of rest and physical activity by including dynamic movements into their warm-up, ensuring that their bodies are appropriately prepared for more intense somatic exercises or conventional workouts. This strategy not only helps to minimize injury, but it also increases training efficiency.

Dynamic Movement Warm-Up

Begin with deep breathing: Before you begin any action, take a minute to focus yourself by breathing deeply into your abdomen. Inhale gently through the nose, allowing the belly to expand before exhaling through the mouth. This technique helps to oxygenate the blood and concentrates the attention on the body's internal status.

Rolls of the Neck and Shoulders

Gently roll the neck in a circular manner, switching directions after a few rotations. Lift the shoulders up towards the ears, then roll them back and down. This helps to relieve stress in the upper body.

Arm swings

Extend your arms out to the sides, swinging them lightly across your body before opening wide again. Gradually increase the pace, using the natural motion to expand the chest and warm up the shoulders.

Hip Circle

Place your hands on your hips and rotate them in a circular manner, rotating clockwise and counterclockwise. This exercise lubricates the hip joints and improves mobility.

Leg swings

Swing one leg forth and backward while holding a steady item for balance. Gradually increase the range of motion. Repeat with the opposite leg. This warms up your leg muscles and hip flexors.

Gentle Squat

Perform a set of soft squats, concentrating on form and the sense of movement in the hips, knees, and ankles. Start with shallow squats and progressively increase depth as your muscles warm up.

Walking lunges

Step forward into a lunge while maintaining the front knee above the ankle. Return to a standing posture with alternating legs. This rapid activity works the primary muscle groups in the legs while boosting heart rate.

Benefits of Dynamic Movement in Somatic Warm-Ups

✓ **Higher Heart Rate and Circulation**: Dynamic motions progressively raise the heart rate, increasing circulation and ensuring that muscles receive an adequate quantity of oxygen and nutrients in preparation for physical activity.

✓ **Increased Muscle Flexibility and Joint Mobility**: These exercises enhance flexibility and mobility by exercising the joints through their whole range of motion, lowering the risk of injury during more demanding activities.

✓ **Improved Coordination and Balance**: Dynamic warm-ups activate both the muscular and neurological systems, which improves coordination and stability. This is especially useful in somatic training, where exact motions and body alignment are essential.

✓ **Increased Body Awareness**: Incorporating mindful movement into the warm-up promotes a greater feeling of bodily awareness. This attentiveness enables people to tune into their bodies' signals and alter their workout accordingly to maximize benefits while minimizing strain.

✓ **Stress Reduction**: Focusing on breath and movement can help to quiet the mind and reduce tension. This mental clarity improves the whole training experience, making it both more effective and pleasurable.

✓ **Preparing for Physical Activity**: These warm-ups operate as a transition between rest and exercise, preparing the body and mind for the physical action ahead. This preparation helps to enhance performance and maximize the advantages of the next workout.

By incorporating dynamic movements into somatic warm-up routines, individuals embarking on a weight loss journey can enjoy a holistic approach to exercise that respects the body's natural rhythms and capabilities. This mindful preparation not only enhances the effectiveness of the workout but also fosters a deeper connection between mind and body, contributing to long-term health and well-being.

Mindfulness Practices for Focus

Incorporating mindfulness techniques into somatic warm-up routines improves attention and connection between mind and body, which is critical for a successful weight reduction journey with somatic exercises. Mindfulness, or being completely present and engaged in the moment without distraction or judgment, can greatly enhance the benefits of physical exercise. Individuals who begin exercises with mindfulness techniques may prepare their minds and bodies for the session ahead, ensuring they get the most out of each action and breath. Here's how to include mindfulness into your somatic warm-up exercises, along with practice instructions and a summary of the advantages.

Start with Deep Breathing

Find a comfortable sitting or standing position. Close your eyes to reduce outside distractions. Concentrate on your breathing, taking slow, deep inhalations through your nose, allowing your chest and belly to fully expand. Exhale gently through your lips, releasing all of the breath and any tension you may be retaining. Repeat for 3-5 minutes, focusing entirely on your breathing patterns. This helps you focus your attention and reduces tension, making it simpler to concentrate on your workout.

Body scan for tension release

After deep breathing, do a mental scan of your body, beginning at the tips of your toes and progressing upward to the crown of your head. Take note of any tense or uncomfortable spots. As you locate these locations, envision breathing into them on each inhale and releasing tension on the exhale. This technique not only improves body awareness but also relaxes the muscles, preparing them for exercise.

Set an Intention for Your Workout

Set a personal objective for your workout while remaining focused on your breath. This might be a goal to be present, listen to your body's needs, or practice self-compassion throughout your session. Setting an intention strengthens your attention and guides your thoughts toward a good and worthwhile aim.

Gentle stretching with mindful attention

Begin your physical warm-up by gently stretching, paying special attention to each action and the sensations it causes in your body. Move slowly and deliberately, taking time to breathe into each stretch. If your mind wanders, gradually return your attention to the sensations of stretching and breathing. This not only warms up the muscles, but it also educates your mind to stay focused on your physical experience.

The Benefits of Mindfulness Practices in Somatic Warm-Up Routines:

1. **Increased focus and concentration**: Starting your workout with mindfulness activities will help free your mind of distractions, allowing you to focus fully on your activity. This increased attention enables improved movement execution, lowering the chance of injury and enhancing the efficacy of your activity.

2. **Improved Body Awareness**: Mindfulness techniques help you become more aware of your body's internal indications and feelings. This enhanced awareness can help you modify your activities to be more successful and supportive of your weight

reduction objectives, ensuring that you are working in harmony with your body rather than pushing it beyond its limitations.

3. **Stress Reduction**: Including mindfulness in your warm-up routine may drastically reduce stress levels. Reduced stress is not just good for mental health; it may also help with physical health by lowering cortisol levels, which can lead to weight gain when increased.

4. **More enjoyment and satisfaction**: Being totally present throughout your workout will undoubtedly increase your appreciation of the activity itself. This favorable experience can boost your motivation and commitment to your workout routine, resulting in long-term weight loss and health benefits.

5. **Improved adaptation to physical stress**: Mindfulness techniques can improve your body's reaction to physical stress, minimizing the risk of overtraining. This is essential for maintaining a consistent fitness regimen without burnout or injury.

Incorporating mindfulness into somatic warm-up activities is an effective method to boost both the mental and physical effects of your exercise. By concentrating on the present moment, you develop a stronger connection with your body, resulting in a more attentive, successful, and joyful approach to weight reduction.

Core Somatic Workouts

Deep Muscle Engagement Exercises

Deep muscular engagement exercises are an essential component of core somatic workouts, especially those geared at weight loss. These movements concentrate on activating and developing the deeper layers of muscular tissue, which are sometimes disregarded in typical training routines. Somatic activities target deep muscles, which not only improve core stability and posture but also metabolic efficiency, resulting in more efficient weight reduction. The descriptions below provide information on several important deep muscle engagement exercises, how to practice them, and the advantages they provide.

The Pelvic Tilt is a basic exercise that works the deep abdominal muscles and lower back. To complete this exercise, lie on your back with knees bent and feet flat on the floor.

- ✓ Inhale deeply, then as you exhale, gently arch your lower back and press it into the floor.

- ✓ Inhale again, and as you exhale, progressively flatten your lower back, moving your belly button closer to your spine.
- ✓ Perform this exercise slowly and deliberately, concentrating on the sense of deep muscular contraction.

Diaphragmatic Breathing is another powerful workout that uses breath work to stimulate the core muscles. Instructions: - Sit or lie down, with one hand on your chest and the other on your abdomen.

- ✓ Inhale deeply through your nose, causing your belly to rise higher than your chest.
- ✓ Exhale slowly through your lips, using your abdominal muscles to force all of the air out.
- ✓ Concentrate on the deep contraction of your core muscles with each exhalation.

The Bridge Lift stresses the lower back, glutes, and hamstrings, as well as deep core stabilizers. To perform this exercise, lie on your back with knees bent, feet flat on the floor, and arms at your sides.

- ✓ Press your feet into the floor and elevate your hips towards the ceiling while maintaining your back straight.

- ✓ Hold the lift at the peak for a few seconds, activating your glutes and core, before gently lowering down.
- ✓ Make sure your deep core muscles are driving the action, and that it is smooth and controlled.

The Leg Slide exercise also works the deep abdominal muscles. The steps are as follows:

- ✓ Lie on your back, legs bent and feet on the floor, with your spine in a neutral posture.
- ✓ Slowly extend one leg at a time, gliding it down the floor before returning to the beginning position.
- ✓ Keep your core muscles engaged and do not lift your lower back off the floor.
- ✓ Alternate legs, ensuring that your deep core muscles are engaged throughout the activity.

These deep muscle engagement workouts provide advantages that go beyond core strength. They improve proprioception, or the feeling of body position, which is essential for doing daily tasks and other exercises more efficiently and with less chance of injury. Improved core stability and strength lead to better posture and can help with lower back discomfort, which is a prevalent problem for many people.

Engaging deep muscle groups can enhance calorie expenditure during and after exercise since they need more energy to activate. This is especially useful for weight loss, since a faster metabolism can aid in fat loss while keeping lean muscle mass.

Finally, the mindfulness component of somatic exercises, which focuses on the internal sensation of movement, encourages a more holistic approach to weight management. It promotes a deeper connection with the body, allowing people to become more aware of their bodily needs and reactions. This understanding may lead to healthier lifestyle choices, better stress management, and a more positive body image, all of which are necessary for long-term weight loss.

Incorporating these deep muscle engagement exercises into a somatic workout program provides a holistic approach to weight management that goes beyond physical activity alone. It represents the combination of mind, body, and spirit, promoting not just physical transformation but also a deep sense of well-being and self-awareness.

Fluid Movement Sequences for Fat Burning

Fluid movement sequences in somatic workouts are designed to enhance body awareness, improve flexibility, and burn fat through gentle, continuous motions that engage multiple muscle groups simultaneously. These sequences are a core component of somatic exercise programs for weight loss, focusing on the quality of movement rather than the intensity or the amount of weight lifted. The emphasis is on how the body feels during the movement, encouraging mindfulness and a deeper connection between the mind and body. This approach can lead to significant fat burning and weight loss over time, as it promotes a more harmonious and efficient way of moving and living.

Benefits of Fluid Movement Sequences

✓ **Enhanced Mind-Body Connection:** Practicing fluid movements helps increase awareness of how the body moves and feels, fostering a deeper connection between physical sensations and mental focus.

✓ **Increased Metabolic Rate**: These sequences engage multiple muscle groups in a continuous flow, which can boost metabolism during and after the workout, aiding in fat burning.

✓ **Improved Flexibility and Mobility**: The gentle, flowing nature of the exercises helps improve joint mobility and muscle flexibility, reducing the risk of injury and enhancing overall movement quality.

✓ **Stress Reduction**: The mindful aspect of fluid movement sequences helps lower stress levels, which is crucial for weight loss, as high stress can lead to emotional eating and weight gain.

✓ **Greater Functional Strength**: These exercises mimic natural body movements, building strength that translates into everyday activities, making daily tasks easier and more efficient.

Instructions for Fluid Movement Sequences

✓ **Start with a Warm-Up**: Begin with 5-10 minutes of gentle stretching or walking in place to prepare your body for movement. Focus on deep breathing to center yourself and enhance body awareness.

✓ **Flow into Cat-Cow Stretches**: On your hands and knees, align your wrists under your shoulders and your knees under your hips. Inhale, arch your back gently, tilt your pelvis up, and look slightly forward for the Cow pose. Exhale, round your spine, tuck your pelvis under, and bring your chin to your chest for the Cat pose. Flow smoothly between these two poses for 2-3 minutes, focusing on the sensation in each movement.

✓ **Transition to Side Stretches**: Stand with feet shoulder-width apart, arms at your sides. Inhale, and as you exhale, gently slide one hand down the side of your leg, bending your torso in that direction. Inhale back to center and repeat on the other side. Continue this side-to-side flow for 2-3 minutes, keeping the movements smooth and fluid.

✓ **Incorporate Arm Sweeps**: In the same standing position, sweep your arms out to the sides and overhead while inhaling, then exhale as you lower them back down. Coordinate the movement with your breath, allowing the arms to flow freely up and down for 2-3 minutes.

✓ **Move into Forward Bends and Rolls**: From standing, inhale and as you exhale, bend forward at the hips, allowing your arms to hang towards the floor. Inhale, slowly rolling up to standing one vertebra at a time, letting your head come up last. Repeat this gentle forward bend and roll up for 3-4 minutes, moving with your breath.

✓ **Finish with a Cool Down**: End your sequence with 5-10 minutes of static stretching or gentle yoga poses to cool down the body. Focus on areas that feel particularly engaged or tight from the workout.

Practicing these fluid movement sequences regularly can significantly contribute to weight loss and overall well-being. The key is to perform the movements mindfully, paying close attention to the sensations in the body and the quality of the breath. This mindful approach not only aids in fat burning but also helps develop a more intuitive relationship with the body, making it easier to maintain a healthy weight and lifestyle. The beauty of fluid movement sequences lies in their simplicity and accessibility, making them a powerful tool for anyone looking to lose weight and improve their health through somatic workouts.

Strength-Building Somatic Routines

Strength-building exercises are essential in somatic workout programs designed for weight reduction, since they combine the concepts of body awareness and mindful movement with the objective of improving muscular strength and composition. These routines differ from standard strength training approaches in that they emphasize movement quality, the link between mind and body, and an understanding of how muscles engage and release during exercise. This novel strategy not only increases physical strength but also improves mental concentration and physiological awareness, providing a comprehensive approach to weight loss and general wellness.

To begin somatic activities that increase strength, you must first establish a foundation of mindfulness and body awareness. Start each session with a few minutes of deep breathing or meditation to help you center yourself and become more aware of your body's feelings and demands. This preliminary stage ensures that your practice is anchored in the present moment and sensitive to the nuances of your body's responses to exercise.

✓ Begin with bodyweight exercises to get acquainted with the feelings of muscular activation. Simple motions like squats, lunges, and push-ups, when done with attention to the breath and movement quality, may greatly improve strength while increasing body awareness.

✓ Use slow and controlled motions, paying close attention to which muscle groups are engaged. For example, during a squat, concentrate on the sensation of your quadriceps, hamstrings, and glutes tightening and relaxing. This mindfulness component transforms each workout into a type of movement meditation, which strengthens the mind-body connection.

✓ Visualization methods can help you deepen muscular involvement. Imagine your muscles extending and contracting with each action, which can improve workout efficacy and enhance neurological connections between your brain and muscles.

✓ Use props like resistance bands or small weights to offer diversity and challenge to your workouts. These tools can help you focus on specific muscle areas while adding resistance in a way that keeps the somatic focus on feeling and control.

- ✓ Include exercises that target all main muscle groups, resulting in a balanced practice that increases overall strength without ignoring any region of the body. Balance and variation are essential for developing a sustainable habit that promotes weight reduction and overall health.
- ✓ Finish each session with a cool-down routine that includes stretching and relaxing activities. This technique helps to release tension that has built up during the workout, aiding healing and preserving the flexibility required for somatic activities.

The advantages of combining strength-building somatic exercises into a weight loss plan are numerous. Physically, these workouts improve muscular tone and metabolic rate, which are both necessary for effective weight reduction. Mentally, focusing on mindfulness and physiological awareness can reduce stress and improve body image, both of which have a substantial influence on weight management. Furthermore, somatic practices that emphasize movement quality and the relationship between mind and body can improve posture, minimize injury risk, and promote general physical functioning.

Individuals can benefit from a multidimensional approach to exercise that recognizes the complexity of the human body by including strength-building somatic activities into a holistic weight reduction regimen. This method not only supports the physical objective of losing weight, but it also builds a stronger connection with the body, improving general well-being and supporting a long-term, healthy lifestyle.

Balancing Exercises for Stability and Core Strength

Balancing exercises are an integral component of core somatic workouts, especially when tailored for weight loss. These exercises not only enhance stability and core strength but also promote mindfulness and body awareness, key principles of somatic practice. Engaging in balancing exercises requires a focus on the present moment and an acute awareness of the body's movements and position in space. This mindful engagement helps to deepen the connection between mind and body, encouraging a more holistic approach to weight loss and overall well-being.

Instructions for Balancing Exercises

Single-Leg Balance

- ✓ Stand on one leg, keeping your weight evenly distributed across the ball and heel.
- ✓ Engage your core and lift your other leg off the ground, bending at the knee.

- ✓ Hold this position for 30 seconds to a minute, focusing on your breathing and the sensations in your standing leg and core.
- ✓ Switch legs and repeat.

Tree Pose (Rossana)

- ✓ Begin standing with feet hip-width apart. Shift your weight onto your right foot.
- ✓ Place the sole of your left foot on your right inner thigh or calf (avoid the knee), toes pointing down.
- ✓ Bring your hands together in front of your chest or raise them above your head, keeping your shoulders down.
- ✓ Hold for 30 seconds to a minute, then switch sides.

Warrior III (Virbhadra's III):

- ✓ Start in a standing position, then extend one leg back as you lean forward, keeping your body and extended leg in a straight line parallel to the floor.
- ✓ Extend your arms forward, beside your head, or back alongside your body for balance.

- ✓ Hold the pose for 15 to 30 seconds, focusing on the engagement of your core and the stability of your supporting leg.

Heel-to-Toe Walk

- ✓ Walk in a straight line, placing the heel of one foot directly in front of the toes of the opposite foot as if walking on a tightrope.
- ✓ Extend your arms sideways to help balance and focus on a point in front of you to maintain stability.
- ✓ Continue for 10 to 20 steps, then reverse direction.

Side Leg Raises

- ✓ Stand with your feet together and a chair or wall beside you for support if needed.
- ✓ Slowly lift one leg to the side, keeping your back straight and your toes facing forward.
- ✓ Hold for a few seconds, then lower back down. Repeat 10-15 times before switching legs.

Benefits of Balancing Exercises for Stability and Core Strength

- ✓ **Enhanced Proprioception:** Balancing exercises improve proprioception, the body's ability to sense its position in space, leading to better movement coordination and agility. This heightened awareness is beneficial for preventing falls and improving performance in other physical activities.

- ✓ **Core Strengthening:** These exercises engage the deep core muscles, including the abdominals, back, and pelvic floor. Strengthening these muscles supports better posture, reduces lower back pain, and enhances the efficiency of movements during other exercises and daily activities.

- ✓ **Increased Caloric Burn:** Balancing exercises require the engagement of multiple muscle groups, increasing the overall energy expenditure even though they might not seem as intense as traditional workouts. This makes them an effective component of a weight loss program.

- ✓ **Mental Focus and Stress Reduction:** The concentration required to maintain balance during these exercises helps to clear the mind, reduce stress, and increase mental focus. The mindful nature of balancing exercises aligns with somatic principles, encouraging a deeper connection between body and mind.

✓ Improved Joint Stability: Regularly performing balancing exercises strengthens the muscles around the joints, improving their stability and reducing the risk of injury. This is particularly important for weight-bearing joints such as the hips, knees, and ankles.

Incorporating balancing exercises into a somatic workout regimen for weight loss offers a multifaceted approach to improving physical health and mental well-being. These exercises not only contribute to a stronger, more stable core and enhanced body awareness but also support the holistic goals of somatic practice, making them a valuable addition to any weight loss or fitness program.

Somatic Cardiovascular Workouts

Heart Rate Elevation with Somatic Movement

Heart rate elevation by somatic movement is a novel and successful technique to cardiovascular exercise, particularly in the setting of weight loss. This technique blends the mindfulness and body awareness inherent in somatic activities with the physiological advantages of higher heart rate seen in more conventional cardiovascular workouts. Individuals can benefit from an exercise that not only burns calories but also improves their connection to their body by engaging in somatic activities that raise the heart rate.

Somatic movement concentrates on the interior experience of movement, stressing the quality of each action and its impact on the body's internal state. When altered to increase the heart rate, these motions become more dynamic, with the focus remaining firmly on physiological sensations and mental states. This conscious approach to boosting cardiovascular activity can result in a more pleasurable, lasting, and successful workout routine, particularly for individuals looking to lose weight.

Instructions for Somatic Cardiovascular Workout

✓ Begin with a Warm-Up: Use gentle somatic activities to stimulate your mind and body. Warm up your muscles and joints by focusing on your breath and moving slowly and deliberately.

✓ Use Dynamic motions: Increase the intensity by include more dynamic, flowing motions. Examples include brisk walking in place, light running, and dynamic stretches that engage the entire body. Keep your motions smooth and prevent any sharp impacts or strains.

✓ Use Imagery and Visualization: As you exercise, imagine your body moving naturally and your heart pounding properly. This mental imagery can strengthen the link between mind and body, enhancing the workout's effects without the need for high-impact movements.

✓ Incorporate Breathing Techniques: Work deep, rhythmic breathing into your actions. For example, time your breathing with your steps or stretches, inhaling deeply as you extend and expelling as you contract. This approach can assist increase your heart rate while keeping you grounded and focused.

✓ Gradually Increase Intensity: As your body warms up, slowly increase the intensity of your motions. This might include a quicker pace, longer strides, or more forceful arm motions. Listen to your body's cues and just push as far as you feel comfortable and sustainable.

✓ Cool Down with moderate Stretching: After reaching the top of your workout, gradually reduce the intensity with moderate somatic stretches. Focus on regions of tension and take deep breaths to help healing and flexibility.

✓ Focus on Your Experience: After your workout, take a few moments of quiet to focus on the feelings in your body and any emotions that developed throughout your practice. This thought can enhance the somatic experience, therefore solidifying the effects of your workout.

Benefit of Heart Rate Elevation with Somatic Movement

1. **Improved Mind-Body Connection**: This method encourages a greater awareness of physical sensations and emotions, so strengthening the mind-body connection and making exercise a more attentive and engaging experience.

2. **Improved Cardiovascular Health**: Raising your heart rate on a regular basis strengthens your heart muscle, improves circulation, and can help lower your risk of heart disease, all of which contribute to good cardiovascular health.

3. **Increased Caloric Burn**: By increasing the heart rate, these workouts can efficiently burn calories, assisting with weight reduction attempts in a more integrated and less mechanical manner than standard cardio exercises.

4. **Reduced tension and Anxiety**: The attentive nature of somatic activities reduces tension and anxiety, providing mental health benefits in addition to physical exercise.

5. **Improved Flexibility and Mobility**: Including dynamic stretches and motions increases flexibility and mobility, lowering the risk of injury and expanding the body's range of motion.

6. **Adaptability and Accessibility**: This approach is easily adaptable to different fitness levels and can be done in a variety of venues with no additional equipment.

7. **Sustainable Exercise Habit**: Because somatic cardiovascular exercises are fun and less demanding, they promote a better long-term approach to fitness and weight management.

Individuals may attain a comprehensive fitness program that promotes both physical and emotional well-being by combining somatic concepts with cardiovascular activities, making it an important part of a weight reduction journey.

High-Intensity Interval Training (HIIT) with a Somatic Twist

High-Intensity Interval Training (HIIT) is a popular workout technique noted for its ability to burn fat, enhance metabolism, and improve cardiovascular health. When paired with a somatic twist, HIIT not only improves physical fitness but also fosters a stronger bond between the mind and body, which is crucial for a comprehensive approach to weight management. This distinct combination incorporates mindfulness, body awareness, and somatic concepts into the dynamic and intense character of HIIT, resulting in a full exercise that addresses both physical and mental well-being.

Instructions for somatic HIIT workouts

- ✓ **Warm-Up with Mindful Breathing**: Start with a 5-minute mindful breathing technique to center yourself and prepare your body and mind for the workout. To promote oxygen flow and body awareness, take deep, diaphragmatic breaths.

✓ **Dynamic Stretching**: For another 5 minutes, do a series of dynamic stretches, focusing on fluid movement and being aware of how each stretch feels in your body. Pay attention to any points of tension or tightness.

✓ **Set Your Intention**: Before beginning the HIIT sequence, take a minute to set a goal for your exercise. This might be expressing thanks for your body's skills or establishing a particular goal for the session.

✓ **HIIT Sequence with Somatic Focus**: Perform each exercise for 30 seconds at high intensity, followed by 30 seconds of mindful movement or static somatic exercises aimed at relaxation and body awareness. Squats, lunges, push-ups, and burpees are examples of dynamic, awareness-based HIIT activities. Incorporate somatic activities such as pelvic tilts, shoulder rolls, or moderate twisting motions into your rest intervals.

✓ **Incorporate Breathing**: Focus on your breathing during the HIIT workout. Try to match your breathing with your motions, expelling during exertion and inhaling during relaxation or less intense periods.

✓ **Cool Down with Somatic Movement**: After finishing the HIIT circuits, take 5-10 minutes to cool down with somatic movements. Choose movements that encourage relaxation and stretch any muscles that were worked hard throughout the session. Concentrate on the feelings in your body and the impact of the workout.

✓ **Reflect and Journal**: Wrap off your workout with a quick session of introspection. Consider keeping a record of your experience, documenting any new feelings or emotions that arise during the workout. Consider your initial aim and the connection you felt with your body during the session.

Benefits of HIIT With a Somatic Twist

✓ **Improved Mind-Body Connection**: By combining somatic concepts into HIIT, people become more aware of their body's signals and wants, resulting in a stronger feeling of body awareness that can improve general well-being.

✓ **Increased Fat Loss and Metabolism**: The afterburn effect of HIIT exercises allows you to burn calories both during and after exercise. The somatic method adds a layer of stress reduction, which can assist reduce cortisol levels and promote fat loss.

✓ **Improved Cardiovascular Health**: This workout enhances heart health by alternating between vigorous bursts of action and recuperation intervals, which effectively tests the cardiovascular system.

✓ **Reduced Stress Levels**: The mindfulness and body awareness techniques embedded in the workout's somatic aspects serve to reduce stress and anxiety, resulting in a more balanced and healthier lifestyle.

✓ **Improved Flexibility and Mobility**: The somatic exercises included in the workout increase flexibility and mobility, lowering the risk of injury and boosting overall physical performance.

✓ **Personalized Workout Experience**: The somatic approach encourages people to listen to their bodies and tailor the intensity and variety of exercises to their own requirements, making the workout extremely customizable and personal.

✓ **Long-term Weight Loss**: By addressing both the physical and psychological components of exercise, this comprehensive HIIT method promotes long-term weight loss and a good connection with physical activity.

Combining HIIT with somatic practices provides a potent weight loss strategy that promotes not only physical health but also mental and emotional well-being. This holistic strategy promotes a balanced and thoughtful attitude to training, resulting in a stronger connection with the body and a more enjoyable and sustainable road to weight loss.

Continuous Movement Flows for Endurance

In the field of somatic training for weight reduction, "Continuous Movement Flows for Endurance" stands out as a critical component, particularly in the cardiovascular workouts portion. This method combines the characteristics of somatic exercise—mindfulness, bodily awareness, and fluid motion—with the endurance-building advantages of cardiovascular training. Unlike typical cardio workouts, which frequently concentrate speed and distance, continuous movement flows emphasize a smooth transition between movements, maintaining a constant rhythm that pushes the heart and lungs while simultaneously fostering a stronger connection with the body.

Instructions for Continuous Movement Flows

- ✓ **Begin with a warm-up**: Use mild motions to arouse the body. Shoulder rolls, neck stretches, and simple side bends improve blood circulation and prepare the body for more active activities.

✓ **Practice Breathing Exercises**: Prior to engaging in more strenuous activities, spend a few minutes focusing on your breath. Deep, diaphragmatic breathing not only oxygenates the blood but also helps to concentrate the mind, allowing you to be more aware of your body's signals during the workout.

✓ **Begin the Flow with Simple motions**: Begin with simple motions like walking in place, waving your arms softly, or stepping sideways. To maintain a high heart rate, move constantly without stopping between changes.

✓ **Gradually Increase Complexity**: As your body warms up, introduce increasingly complicated motions such as squats, lunges, and arm reach. Ensure that each action flows into the next without pausing, resulting in a dance-like sequence that keeps the body engaged and the mind concentrated.

✓ **Incorporate multi-directional activities**: Include activities that involve turning, twisting, and bending to activate various muscle groups and improve agility and coordination. This variation not only increases the efficacy of the workout, but it also makes it more fascinating and pleasurable.

✓ **Maintain Mindfulness**: Throughout the flow, keep your attention on your body's internal experiences. Consider the sense of your muscles contracting, your heart pounding, and your breath matching with your motions. The awareness factor distinguishes somatic cardiovascular workouts from standard cardio routines.

✓ **Cool Down and Reflect**: Finish your workout with a cool-down phase that includes slower, methodical movements and stretches. This is the moment to reflect on your experience, recognizing any changes in your energy, emotions, or physical status since you started.

Benefits of Continuous Movement Flows for Endurance

✓ **Improved Cardiovascular Health**: These fluxes raise heart rate and respiration, which improves cardiovascular endurance and efficiency. Over time, this can lead to lower resting heart rates and better circulation.

✓ **Increased Metabolic Rate**: Continuous activity challenges the body in a way that increases metabolism not just during the workout but also for hours afterward, assisting in weight reduction.

- ✓ **Improved Body Awareness**: The emphasis on fluid motion and awareness allows practitioners to establish a stronger connection with their bodies, which improves coordination and movement efficiency in everyday life.

- ✓ **Tension Reduction**: The contemplative nature of continuous flows can assist alleviate tension. The repetitive quality of the motions, along with concentrated breathing, calms the nervous system.

- ✓ **Flexibility and Strength Gains**: Stretching and muscular engagement are common features of these flows, which can help develop flexibility and strength, particularly in the core and stabilizer muscles.

- ✓ **Improved Mental concentration**: The demand to concentrate on the flow of motions improves mental concentration and clarity, which may be applied beyond the exercise to daily tasks.

- ✓ **Adaptability**: Continuous movement flows are readily tweaked to accommodate varied fitness levels, making them accessible to beginners while remaining demanding for more advanced athletes.

Individuals who include continuous movement flows into a somatic training routine for weight reduction can have a complete exercise experience that improves not just physical health but also mental and emotional well-being. This strategy is a welcome departure from standard cardiovascular training, providing a road to endurance and strength that is both effective and genuinely rewarding.

Mind-Body Connection

Techniques to Enhance Mindfulness during Exercise

Practicing mindfulness while exercising elevates the workout experience from a typical activity to a deeply personal journey of mind-body connection. This technique, which is key to somatic exercises for weight reduction, emphasizes the quality of each action, urging people to be acutely aware of their bodies. Individuals may build a state of mindfulness by paying close attention to the sensations that emerge during exercise, such as the rhythm of breathing, the alignment of the spine, or the activation of muscles, which not only improves their workout but also helps them lose weight. This increased awareness aids in identifying the body's signs of exhaustion and fullness, resulting in improved control of physical activity and eating habits.

One effective way to promote mindfulness while exercise is to start each session with a moment of calm. Taking the time to concentrate oneself before beginning to exercise might help establish a mental space dedicated to the training. This technique includes deep breathing and creating an objective for the exercise, which might be as simple as concentrating on the breath during the workout or being patient with oneself. Such objectives serve as anchors, bringing the mind back to the present moment whenever it wanders, thereby incorporating mindfulness into physical action.

Breath practice is another key component of improving awareness when exercising. Concentrating on the breath helps to integrate the mind and body, directing movement and establishing a rhythmical flow of exercises. Individuals may enrich their somatic experience, boost their stamina, and make their exercises more efficient by noticing their natural intake and exhale and coordinating breath with action. This mindful breathing also helps to navigate the intensity of the activity, ensuring that one does not push past their physical limits, which is critical for preventing injury and maintaining long-term weight reduction.

Body scanning is a mindfulness-based approach that may be smoothly incorporated into workout programs. This is mentally scanning the entire body from head to toe, recording any feelings, tensions, or discomforts without judgment. Body scanning allows people to become more aware of their physical state, allowing them to alter their movements to better fit their body's demands. This practice not only strengthens the mind-body connection, but it also encourages self-care, which is necessary for a good weight reduction journey.

Visualization methods are also important for maintaining mindfulness when exercising. Imagining the muscles moving and the body strengthening may increase mental involvement in the workout, making it more effective and pleasurable. Visualization not only enhances motivation, but it also aids in obtaining a higher level of attention and focus, which are essential components of a mindful workout. Visualizing desirable outcomes, such as a healthier, stronger body, allows people to stay connected to their long-term weight reduction objectives, making each activity feel more significant.

Incorporating variation into your training regimen is another method to stay alert and focused. Trying diverse types of somatic activities, such as yoga, Pilates, tai chi, or dance, can provide fresh sensations and challenges, keeping the mind from going into autopilot during workouts. This diversity keeps the mind interested and attentive, completely experiencing each action and its effect on the body. Such diversity not only eliminates boredom, but also allows people to explore other elements of their physically, which may be quite fulfilling and beneficial to weight reduction.

Finally, ending each workout with a moment of reflection strengthens the mind-body connection. Taking a few moments to focus on the sensations felt during the workout, as well as the obstacles and accomplishments, can help to reinforce mindfulness. This meditation period can also be used to express thanks to the body for its power and resilience, therefore building a healthy relationship with one's physical self. Through these strategies, mindfulness is woven into the fabric of exercise, transforming it into a holistic practice that promotes not just weight reduction but also general health.

Using Visualization for Weight Loss

Visualization, a powerful technique in the domain of somatic training, uses the mind-body link to promote weight reduction. This strategy entails constructing vivid mental representations of desired results, such as obtaining a specific body weight or effectively conducting physical workouts. Individuals who use their imaginations might increase their enthusiasm and devotion to their weight reduction quest. Visualization not only prepares the mind for achievement, but it also changes the body's physiological responses, which are aligned with one's objectives. As part of a somatic workout, visualization helps to strengthen the connection between mental intents and physical activities, making the weight reduction process more integrated and meaningful.

To incorporate visualization into somatic workouts, focus on the sensory and emotional sensations involved with achieving weight reduction objectives. For example, envisioning yourself moving more freely and easily might elicit feelings of exhilaration and anticipation. This method helps people to see and feel the advantages of weight loss, which boosts their drive. Individuals who clearly see themselves as healthier and more active might create a good emotional and psychological state that encourages persistent effort toward their goals.

Visualization is also important in conquering the problems and barriers that come on the weight reduction journey. When faced with a challenge, people might utilize visualization to remind themselves of their goals and the reasons for their dedication. Visualizing previous achievements or favorable results can boost confidence and resilience, allowing people to approach setbacks with a more constructive and hopeful attitude. This mental rehearsal prepares the brain for success, making it simpler to stay focused even when confronted with temptation or difficulty.

Beyond motivation and resilience, visualization can improve the efficiency of physical exercise, which is an essential component of somatic exercises. Individuals who mentally rehearse certain actions or activities can enhance their physical performance and skill. This mental exercise engages the same cerebral pathways as physical exertion, resulting in increased strength, coordination, and endurance. As a result, visualization not only helps with the psychological components of weight reduction, but it also directly adds to physical growth and competence.

The use of visualization in somatic workouts highlights the overall aspect of weight loss. It recognizes that reaching a healthy weight entails more than simply physical changes; it necessitates a shift in how people see and connect to their bodies. Visualization promotes a good and empowered mental picture, resulting in a more loving and respectful connection with the body. This shift in viewpoint is critical for long-term success because it shifts the emphasis away from external measurements of development and toward a better understanding of the body's potential and value.

Furthermore, visualizing promotes stress reduction, which is essential for successful weight loss. Stress is known to sabotage weight reduction efforts by inducing bad eating habits and delaying metabolism. Individuals can reduce the effects of stress on their bodies by using visualization methods that promote relaxation and mental clarity. Individuals can maintain a more balanced and healthier attitude to weight reduction by visualizing tranquil and serene surroundings or utilizing guided imagery to easily manage difficult situations.

Finally, using imagination during somatic workouts is a highly effective weight reduction method. It takes advantage of the fundamental link between mind and body, providing a means to not only envisioning achievement but also embodying it. Individuals who use visualization can boost their drive, conquer obstacles, increase physical performance, cultivate a good body image, and reduce stress. This multimodal approach emphasizes the significance of addressing both the emotional and physical components of weight reduction, resulting in a full and holistic road to reaching health and wellness objectives.

The Role of Interoception in Fitness and Weight Management

Interoception, or awareness of the body's internal condition, is an important component in understanding and maintaining fitness and weight. This inner awareness includes the ability to notice bodily feelings like hunger, thirst, heart rate, and even the movement of the diaphragm when breathing. Interoception is important in somatic exercises and weight control because it allows people to listen in to their bodies' cues, building a stronger connection between mind and body. This link is important for detecting the body's requirements, which leads to more conscious decisions about nutrition, exercise, and overall well-being.

Somatic exercise, which focuses on interior perception and movement sensation, directly engages and improves interoception. By emphasizing how actions feel rather than how they seem, these exercises promote a shift from outward validation to interior sensation. This change is critical for weight control because it shifts the emphasis away from the scale and toward a more comprehensive view of health. Enhanced interoception through somatic activities enables people to distinguish between actual physical hunger and emotional eating, resulting in healthier eating habits and more successful weight control.

Furthermore, interoceptive awareness developed by somatic workouts might lead to better stress management, which is critical in weight management. Stress has been shown to influence food patterns, exercise motivation, and general health. Individuals can learn to notice and decrease stress-related physiological signs through methods such as mindful breathing and body scanning. This understanding can help prevent stress-related overeating and promote choices that support fitness and weight management objectives, emphasizing the link between mental and physical health.

Interoception can help improve physical performance and prevent injuries. Individuals who have a comprehensive awareness of the body's signals can adapt their routines to avoid overexertion and identify early symptoms of damage. This sensitivity enables more tailored and successful training programs, which are vital for long-term weight loss and general health. Somatic exercises, which focus on soft, focused movements, are especially good in developing this acute sense of physical awareness.

Interoception is very important in determining motivation and enjoyment of physical activity. A strong mind-body connection, developed via interoception-enhancing activities, may elevate exercise from a drudgery to an enjoyable pastime. This change is critical for long-term participation in fitness routines because it fosters a good attitude toward exercise and a desire to maintain an active lifestyle, both of which are essential components of successful weight control.

Furthermore, somatic workouts can help enhance interoceptive awareness, resulting in a more loving and accepting connection with the body. This psychological advantage is important for weight control because it challenges cultural standards and self-critical attitudes that can lead to unhealthy behavior. Individuals are more likely to stick to their fitness and weight reduction objectives if they are surrounded by a friendly and nonjudgmental environment.

To summarize, including interoceptive awareness into fitness and weight control via somatic exercises provides a complete strategy that addresses the physical, emotional, and psychological elements of health. This method not only promotes good weight control, but it also leads to a higher sense of well-being and a more harmonious relationship with one's body. Individuals who are more aware of their internal states are better able to make educated, thoughtful decisions that support their fitness and weight management objectives, demonstrating the significant influence of the mind-body link on overall health.

Nutrition and Somatic Exercise

Eating Mindfully to Support Weight Loss

Eating mindfully is a revolutionary method that is well aligned with the ideas of somatic exercises, emphasizing the need of listening to the body's messages to aid in weight reduction. This practice entails giving complete attention to the sensation of eating and drinking, both within and outside of the body. It promotes an understanding of the physical and sensory sensations linked with food, such as taste, smell, and texture, as well as the emotional emotions they may elicit. Mindful eating enables people to detect actual hunger and satiety signals, which helps them avoid overeating and makes it simpler to make better meal choices that support their weight reduction objectives.

Incorporating mindful eating into a weight reduction strategy can result in a greater appreciation for food, converting it from a thoughtless act to a purposeful and joyful experience. Slowing down and enjoying each mouthful typically results in people needing less food to feel content, allowing them to gradually reduce their calorie consumption without feeling deprived. This moves away from automatic eating behaviors can have a substantial influence on a person's ability to lose weight and keep it off over time. Mindful eating techniques prohibit multitasking during meals, such as watching TV or scrolling through social media, as this can lead to distracted eating and a dissociation from the body's hunger and fullness signals.

The concepts of mindful eating go beyond the act of eating itself, advocating a more holistic view of food as nourishment for the body and spirit. This viewpoint promotes a healthy relationship with food, in which decisions are focused on nutritional worth and personal enjoyment rather than emotional comfort or dietary constraints. Individuals who learn to connect with food in this way can break the cycle of yo-yo dieting and build a sustainable attitude to eating that promotes weight loss and general well-being.

Mindful eating also compliments the somatic workout approach to weight reduction by promoting an awareness of the body's requirements. Just as somatic exercises increase awareness of the body's internal states and subtle signals, mindful eating techniques help people realize when they are eating out of habit, boredom, or emotional discomfort rather than genuine hunger. This understanding can result in more deliberate eating behaviors, in which food is ingested to nourish the body and promote physical activity rather than to satisfy emotional cravings.

Mindful nutrition may also improve the efficiency of somatic workouts by keeping the body properly fed and nourished. Understanding and reacting to the body's dietary demands ensures that individuals have the energy and endurance to complete their activities, aiding weight reduction and boosting muscle repair and growth. The symbiotic link between mindful eating and physical activity is essential for developing a balanced and healthy lifestyle that promotes long-term weight management.

Furthermore, mindful eating promotes a nonjudgmental attitude toward food and body image, which is essential for developing self-esteem and motivation during the weight reduction process. By eliminating guilt and shame from the eating experience, people may build a more loving and supportive connection with their bodies. This positive mentality is critical for overcoming setbacks and staying dedicated to health objectives, therefore mindful eating is a key component of a successful weight reduction plan.

Mindful eating is an essential component of the somatic exercise approach to weight reduction, providing a pathway to a healthier and more harmonious connection with food and the body. Mindful eating habits promote long-term weight loss and improve general health and well-being by instilling awareness, appreciation, and a strong connection to the physical and emotional elements of food. This comprehensive approach not only supports in attaining weight reduction objectives but also increases the quality of life, making it a beneficial practice for anybody wishing to better their health via mindfulness and somatic exercise.

Nutritional Tips to Complement Your Somatic Workout

Nutritional practices are essential for maximizing the advantages of somatic exercises, particularly when weight loss is the aim. Somatic exercises, which emphasize mindfulness and bodily awareness, provide a unique opportunity to better understand and nurture the body. This idea also applies to nutrition, where the kind of food delivered to the body affects its performance, recuperation, and general well-being. Individuals who practice mindful eating can supplement their somatic practices by ensuring that their bodies are fully fed to sustain the moderate, yet deep, physical activities required.

Mindful eating is an important nutritional suggestion for individuals who participate in somatic workouts. It entails giving complete attention to the sensation of eating and drinking, both within and outside the body. Mindful eating promotes an awareness of the physical and emotional signals that influence eating behaviors, allowing people to make more mindful food choices that support their weight reduction and wellness objectives. This practice adheres to the concepts of somatic exercise by encouraging a closer connection with the body's requirements, satiety signals, and reactions to various meals.

Hydration is extremely important in supporting somatic exercises. The body's requirement for water is increased during exercise to maintain peak performance and speed up recovery. Adequate hydration promotes fluidity of movement, which is essential for somatic workouts, as well as effective nutrition delivery to cells, waste disposal, and body temperature control. Drinking water on a regular basis throughout the day, particularly before and after somatic activities, ensures that the body operates properly and benefits in weight control by reducing overeating, which is sometimes confused with thirst.

A balanced diet rich in complete foods is another important nutritional suggestion that supports somatic workouts. Whole foods, such as fruits and vegetables, whole grains, lean proteins, and healthy fats, supply the body with a wide range of nutrients required for energy, muscle repair, and general health. These nutrients promote the body's natural healing processes, improving the advantages of somatic therapies that attempt to relieve tension and restore equilibrium. A diet based on whole foods is also consistent with mindful eating concepts, fostering a better appreciation for the quality and origin of the foods ingested.

The timing of meals and snacks relative to somatic training sessions can have a substantial influence on performance and recuperation. Consuming a short, balanced meal or snack high in carbs and protein before an exercise helps give the energy required for the activity, while having a comparable snack afterward promotes muscle repair and energy replacement. This strategy guarantees that the body has enough food to participate in somatic practices successfully and that recovery is maximized, resulting in weight loss and improved physical fitness.

The need of anti-inflammatory nutrients in a diet to supplement somatic exercises cannot be emphasized. Chronic inflammation can impede the body's healing process and harm general health, potentially jeopardizing weight loss attempts. Consuming anti-inflammatory foods such as omega-3-rich fish, nuts, seeds, leafy greens, and berries might help the body's natural healing capabilities. This nutritional approach is especially useful when combined with somatic exercises, which promote healing and recovery by lowering stress and tension in the body.

Finally, listening to the body's hunger and fullness cues is a practice that complements both somatic exercise and nutritional health. Somatic activities improve body awareness, particularly the capacity to detect genuine hunger cues and fullness. Individuals can avoid overeating by paying attention to these signals and choosing foods that truly meet their nutritional needs while also supporting their weight loss journey. This practice of attunement ensures that nutrition and somatic exercise work in tandem to promote health, well-being, and a balanced approach to weight management. Together, these dietary techniques not only improve the physical advantages of somatic exercises, but also encourage a holistic approach to health that takes into account the complicated relationships between the body, mind, and the sustenance they receive.

Hydration and Its Importance in Somatic Practice

Hydration is critical for increasing the effectiveness of somatic practices, especially when combined with a weight loss regimen. At its core, somatic exercise emphasizes the mind-body connection, using internal awareness to guide movements and breath. Water, the essence of life, is essential in this process because it enhances the body's natural ability to communicate and function properly. Adequate hydration ensures that every cell, tissue, and organ in the body functions properly, which supports the nuanced bodily awareness that somatic workouts seek to cultivate.

Water's role in somatic weight loss practice goes beyond simple hydration; it is essential for maintaining movement fluidity and muscle flexibility. Somatic exercises frequently involve gentle, flowing movements that require the muscles to be hydrated and flexible. Dehydration, on the other hand, can cause muscle stiffness and reduced elasticity, limiting the body's ability to perform somatic movements comfortably and increasing the risk of injury. Thus, staying hydrated is critical for facilitating the smooth, mindful movements that define somatic practice.

Furthermore, hydration affects metabolic processes that are important for weight loss. Water plays an important role in converting stored fat into energy, which is necessary for weight loss. Individuals can improve their metabolism and manage their weight more effectively by staying hydrated. Somatic practice, with its emphasis on body awareness, provides an opportunity to tune into the body's hydration signals, promoting a more intuitive approach to drinking water and recognizing its importance in energy production and weight loss.

Hydration also influences concentration and mental clarity, both of which are essential in somatic exercises. These practices necessitate a high level of mental concentration because they involve focusing on bodily sensations, movements, and breathing exercises. A well-hydrated brain performs better, increasing focus and the ability to maintain mindfulness during somatic sessions. This increased awareness not only improves the quality of the workout, but it also strengthens the mind-body connection that is central to somatic philosophy.

Hydration is essential for recovery because it helps flush out toxins and facilitates muscle repair. Somatic workouts, while typically low-impact, still work the muscles and tissues, necessitating recovery. Water aids in the transport of nutrients to cells and the removal of waste products, thereby speeding up the recovery process. This is especially important in weight loss situations where regular exercise is part of the plan. Adequate hydration allows the body to recover efficiently, allowing for consistent participation in somatic practices with minimal downtime.

Hydration also has a direct effect on appetite and satiety, which are important factors in weight management. Often, the body misinterprets dehydration signals for hunger, resulting in increased food intake when what it really needs is water. Individuals who stay properly hydrated can better distinguish between true hunger cues and thirst cues, thereby preventing overeating. This understanding of the body's signals is aided by somatic practice, which cultivates a keen awareness of bodily needs, including hydration.

Finally, the ritual of hydrating can become a mindful practice in and of itself, reflecting the somatic emphasis on intentionality and presence. Hydration in somatic workouts promotes a holistic approach to health, viewing water not only as a physical necessity, but also as a nourishing act that aids the body's journey through movement and transformation. This holistic approach, which combines hydration and somatic exercises, provides a comprehensive path to weight loss that recognizes the body's interconnected needs for movement, awareness, and nourishment.

Recovery and Relaxation Techniques

Somatic Practices for Cool Down

Somatic practices for cooling down are essential in any weight loss journey because they focus on the body's recovery and relaxation following exercise. These practices are intended to restore awareness to the body, allowing for a smooth transition from the intensity of a workout to a state of rest. Somatic cool-down exercises teach people how to release tension, reduce muscle soreness, and improve flexibility, all of which are essential for sticking to an exercise routine. The mindful approach of somatic practices encourages participants to tune into their bodies, identifying areas of tightness or discomfort and using gentle movement to relieve them.

Focused breathing is a key component of the somatic cool down. Deep, controlled breathing helps to oxygenate the muscles, which aids recovery and reduces stress. This method of breathing not only promotes physical relaxation but also mental calmness, preparing the body and mind for the end of a workout session. Individuals who pay attention to the rhythm and depth of their breath can strengthen their connection to their bodies, promoting a sense of peace and well-being that aids weight loss efforts by reducing stress-induced eating habits.

Progressive muscle relaxation is another somatic technique that helps you cool down. It entails tensing and then relaxing various muscle groups, which can aid in identifying tension points in the body. This practice not only helps to relieve muscle tension, but it also teaches the body to recognize and distinguish between sensations of tension and relaxation. Over time, this awareness can lead to more efficient muscle recovery and a lower risk of injury, both of which are necessary for maintaining an active lifestyle conducive to weight loss.

Gentle stretching is an essential component of somatic cool-down practices. Unlike static stretching, somatic stretching emphasizes movement and awareness. It encourages people to stretch in a way that feels good for their bodies, moving slowly and deliberately. This method allows for a more thorough release of tight muscles and increases overall flexibility, which can improve performance in future workouts and daily activities. The mindful nature of somatic stretching strengthens the connection between mind and body, reinforcing a holistic approach to weight loss.

Body scanning is a technique used in somatic practices to promote mindfulness and relaxation. It entails mentally scanning the body from head to toe, taking note of any sensations, tensions, or emotions that arise. This practice can be especially beneficial after a workout because it allows people to become more aware of how their bodies feel and where they should focus their recovery efforts. Individuals who incorporate body scanning into their cool-down routine can address areas of discomfort before they cause pain or injury, thereby supporting continued physical activity and weight loss.

Somatic cool-down practices also incorporate visualization techniques. Individuals are encouraged to imagine their muscles relaxing and all tension melting away. This mental imagery has a significant impact on the body's ability to relax and recover. Visualization not only aids in physical relaxation but also in emotional and mental recovery, reducing anxiety and stress that can stymie weight loss efforts. Individuals can use visualization to end their workout in a peaceful, restorative manner, reinforcing the positive experiences associated with exercise.

Incorporating somatic practices into the cool-down phase is about more than just physical recovery; it's about fostering a holistic sense of well-being that aids in weight loss. These practices teach people to listen to their bodies, meet their needs, and recognize their efforts. This respectful and mindful approach to exercise and recovery has the potential to improve the long-term viability and enjoyment of weight loss. Individuals who incorporate somatic cool-down techniques can improve their physical and mental recovery, paving the way for a healthier, more balanced approach to achieving their weight loss goals.

Stress Reduction Techniques

Stress has a substantial negative impact on weight reduction and general well-being, frequently defeating efforts to live a healthier lifestyle. The somatic workout method, based on bodily awareness and mindfulness, offers a powerful antidote to stress through a variety of reduction approaches. These techniques not only help with weight reduction by addressing one of the most prevalent hurdles, but they also improve recuperation and relaxation, which are essential for a healthy body and mind. Individuals may engage their parasympathetic nervous system, the body's rest and digest response, which is vital for stress reduction and recovery, by learning to listen to its subtle cues and respond with conscious activity.

Deep breathing exercises, which are central to somatic therapies, are an effective stress-reduction technique. Individuals can avoid the stress-induced fight or flight reaction by focusing on deep, deliberate breaths, which lowers cortisol levels and reduces overall stress. This technique not only promotes instant relaxation, but it also encourages a more conscious attitude to food and physical exercise, which supports long-term weight reduction attempts. The regular pattern of deep breathing promotes a meditative state, allowing for a stronger connection between mind and body, which is useful in identifying and managing stress causes.

Progressive muscular relaxation (PMR) shows how somatic workouts reduce stress. This technique includes tensing and then releasing various muscle groups to increase awareness of physical tension and relaxation. PMR can be especially useful for people who carry tension in their muscles, resulting in persistent soreness or stiffness that can impede effective exercise and weight reduction. Individuals who practice PMR on a daily basis can improve their capacity to relax both mind and body, resulting in better sleep quality and recovery, both of which are essential components of a weight reduction routine.

Body scanning is another somatic practice that promotes relaxation while supplementing established weight loss measures. Individuals use this exercise to deliberately focus on different portions of their bodies, recording sensations without judgment. This mindfulness practice promotes calm and relaxation, which reduces stress and its negative consequences on weight control. Body scanning not only helps to discover areas of stress and discomfort, but it also fosters a comprehensive sense of well-being, making it simpler to adopt healthy lifestyle habits.

Visualization methods, which are frequently used in somatic workouts, are also effective in stress reduction. Individuals might produce a mood of calm and happiness by envisioning tranquil sights or seeing their goals being achieved. This mental rehearsal can reduce stress, increase motivation, and strengthen the mental resilience required to stick to a weight reduction strategy. Visualization not only aids in the psychological elements of weight control, but it also improves the physical healing process by encouraging a good and peaceful mental state.

Mindful movement, an essential component of somatic exercises, provides a dynamic technique to relieve stress while engaging in physical activity. Rather than focusing on the intensity or consequence of exercise, mindful movement focuses the sensation of movement itself, which promotes feelings of joy and freedom. This method may turn exercise from a stressful duty to a source of relaxation and enjoyment, therefore aiding weight reduction attempts by making physical activity more desirable and sustainable.

Finally, including somatic techniques into everyday routines provides a solid basis for long-term stress management and weight control. Individuals may create a toolkit for dealing with stress in a comprehensive and successful way by using strategies including deep breathing, PMR, body scanning, visualization, and mindful movement. These activities not only help with immediate stress relief, but they also enable people to take a balanced approach to weight loss, emphasizing the necessity of recuperation and relaxation. Somatic workouts make the weight loss journey more harmonic and durable, and stress management is essential for reaching and maintaining optimal health.

Deep Relaxation and Recovery Exercises

Deep relaxation and recuperation exercises are essential components of somatic workouts for weight reduction, serving as the yin to the yang of physical activity. These techniques are not only for taking a break; they are essential to the process of reducing weight in a healthy and sustainable way. Individuals can dramatically improve their body's ability to recover from exercise, manage stress, and contribute to efficient weight control by practicing techniques such as progressive muscle relaxation, guided imagery, and deep diaphragmatic breathing.

Progressive muscle relaxation, a technique that includes tensing and then releasing each muscle area, is especially effective after dynamic movements in somatic workouts. This practice not only relieves muscular tension and reduces physical stress, but it also has a significant relaxing impact on the mind. Individuals can relieve accumulated stress by carefully going through their bodies, which is a typical obstacle to weight reduction since tension causes cortisol production and subsequent weight gain. This technique encourages a deeper connection with the body, allowing people to perceive and respond to their bodily state, resulting in a more holistic approach to weight loss.

Guided imagery, another effective deep relaxation technique, supports somatic activities by facilitating mental and emotional recovery. Visualizing tranquil images or optimistic outcomes can greatly reduce tension, which aids weight reduction attempts by decreasing the risk of stress-induced eating. This mental exercise improves the mind-body connection, which is essential for somatic practice, allowing people to visualize their objectives and create a sense of serenity that benefits in healing and general well-being.

Deep diaphragmatic breathing is essential for relaxation and recuperation during somatic exercises. Slow, deep breaths can stimulate the parasympathetic nervous system, promoting relaxation and digestion. This not only helps with post-exercise recovery, but it also regulates appetite and reduces emotional eating. Mastering this type of breathing improves oxygen flow and nutrition delivery to muscles, hastening recuperation and ensuring that the body is prepared for the next somatic activity.

Mindfulness meditation promotes deeper relaxation and recuperation. Individuals participating in somatic workouts for weight reduction might create an awareness that extends beyond the workout itself by examining thoughts and feelings without judgment. This awareness can lead to healthier eating habits since one becomes more aware of hunger and satiety signals, making them less likely to participate in mindless eating. Furthermore, mindfulness meditation can enhance sleep quality, which is important for weight reduction and recovery since insufficient sleep impairs the body's capacity to mend and maintain a healthy weight.

Yoga and gentle stretching during the recovery period of a somatic training regimen provide an additional layer of relaxation and healing. These techniques increase flexibility, reduce discomfort, and promote circulation, which aids in the elimination of toxins and accelerates muscle healing. Slow, purposeful movements in yoga and stretching, along with deep breathing, help to enhance the mind-body connection, fostering a meditative state that aids in weight reduction by increasing mental clarity and emotional balance.

Finally, using autogenic training, a self-relaxation approach that involves silently repeating affirmations to generate physiological sensations of warmth and heaviness, can be especially beneficial following somatic workouts. This strategy improves mental health and stress management, which are important aspects of weight loss. Autogenic training, which reduces stress and increases a sense of control over one's body, compliments the somatic approach to weight loss, which focuses on building harmony and balance within the body.

These deep relaxation and recovery exercises complement the somatic workout experience by addressing key components such as stress management, muscular recovery, and emotional well-being. They ensure that weight reduction is more than just burning calories via physical exercise; it is also about nourishing the body and mind, resulting in a long-term route to health and fitness

Challenges and Solutions

Overcoming Common Obstacles in Somatic Exercise

Starting a journey with somatic exercise for weight reduction poses unique obstacles since it necessitates a transition from typical exercise attitudes to ones that stress inward awareness and mindfulness. One major barrier is the difficulty of tuning into one's own bodily signals. Many people are used to ignoring or overcoming body feelings, particularly during activity. The approach is to begin with easy mindfulness techniques like focused breathing and body scans, then progressively improve awareness to internal cues. Over time, this increased awareness fosters a stronger connection with the body, allowing people to do somatic activities more efficiently.

Another difficulty is the assumption that somatic activities are insufficiently intense to aid in weight loss. This mindset may discourage people from completely committing to the practice. Somatic activities, while often moderate, deeply activate muscles and enhance metabolic function. Educating oneself about the physiological advantages of these exercises, such as how they improve muscular tone, flexibility, and stress reduction—all of which are essential components of weight loss—can inspire people to incorporate somatic practices into their daily lives.

Resistance to slow-paced activities is also prevalent, since many people equate weight loss with high-intensity exercise. The slower pace of somatic exercises is intended to promote body awareness and limit the chance of injury, which is critical for long-term weight loss. To overcome this obstacle, people might progressively include somatic exercises into their regular routines, valuing the balance of high-intensity workouts and contemplative movements. This combination provides a holistic approach to exercise, addressing both physical and mental wellness.

A lack of apparent success might be disappointing for people who use somatic activities to lose weight. Unlike traditional workouts, where progress can be quantified in pounds lifted or kilometers ran, the advantages of somatic exercises are frequently felt before they are seen. Keeping a notebook to track changes in feelings, mood, and bodily awareness can help people realize and appreciate the small but major effects of their practice. This introspective approach promotes patience and tenacity while emphasizing the underlying benefits of somatic activities.

Another problem is fitting somatic exercises into a hectic lifestyle. Making time for mindfulness and movement may seem difficult. However, somatic activities may be easily integrated into everyday life. Simple techniques, like mindful walking or aware stretching during breaks, can have a huge impact. The idea is to see somatic exercise as an enriching component of daily life that improves the quality of both movement and rest.

For others, the solitary nature of somatic exercises may feel lonely, particularly for people who thrive in group training environments. Building a community of like-minded people who are also interested in somatic practices may be a source of support and inspiration. Online forums, local classes, and group sessions allow you to interact, share experiences, and learn from others. This sense of community not only alleviates feelings of loneliness, but it also deepens the somatic exercise journey with shared experiences and support.

Finally, navigating the huge diversity of somatic exercises accessible might be daunting. Individuals may struggle to select techniques that best meet their needs and aspirations if they are not given clear direction. Seeking out credible sources, publications, and teachers that specialize in somatic exercise can help give guidance and organization. Personalized coaching or seminars geared to weight reduction objectives can also make practices more successful and pleasant. Individuals who address these obstacles with educated tactics and answers may fully embrace somatic exercise as a strong weight reduction tool, opening the door to a more connected and conscious approach to health and fitness.

Addressing Plateaus in Weight Loss

Many people suffer weight reduction plateaus, which are defined as a time of no noticeable progress while keeping a balanced diet and exercise plan. This standstill may be unpleasant and demotivating, prompting some people to discontinue their weight-loss efforts entirely. However, somatic exercises provide a more nuanced approach to overcome these plateaus by establishing a stronger connection between the mind and body, which can uncover underlying difficulties that standard approaches may overlook.

One of the most common reasons of weight reduction plateaus is the body's adaptability to routine. Somatic exercises, which focus on internal awareness and movement exploration, offer a chance to add variation to an exercise routine. Individuals may push their bodies in new ways by adjusting their routines based on how their bodies feel throughout various motions. This not only helps to break through physical plateaus, but it also maintains the workout experience interesting and engaging, lowering the danger of burnout.

Stress is another key element that might impede weight reduction efforts. Somatic techniques, such as conscious breathing and gentle movement, can effectively lower stress levels. Lower stress levels are connected with reduced cortisol production, a hormone that, when excessive, can cause weight gain or a weight loss stall. Incorporating somatic activities into everyday routines can help to build a more balanced internal environment, which is more beneficial to weight loss.

Plateaus in weight reduction are frequently exacerbated by emotional eating, in which people resort to food for consolation rather than nutrition. Somatic workouts assist practitioners create a conscious relationship with their bodies, allowing them to understand emotional cues that cause overeating. Individuals who learn to detect and handle these cues via somatic awareness can build healthy coping methods that do not rely on food, which will help them achieve their weight reduction objectives.

Sleep quality, which is often disregarded in typical weight reduction regimens, is critical for breaking through plateaus. Somatic activities, particularly those aimed at relaxation and stress reduction, might enhance sleep quality. Better sleep promotes weight reduction by modulating hormones like ghrelin and leptin, which govern hunger and fat storage. Integrating somatic activities into evening rituals can help people relax and prepare for a good night's sleep, which can help them lose weight.

Another strategy to overcoming weight reduction plateaus is to examine and alter food habits. Somatic awareness promotes a more intuitive approach to eating by encouraging people to listen to their bodies' hunger and fullness cues. This can lead to more conscious food choices and portion sizes, bringing eating habits closer to the body's real demands. Over time, this mindful eating technique can help break through weight reduction plateaus by limiting overeating and promoting a healthy diet.

Finally, overcoming a weight reduction stall might provide a chance for personal growth and more body respect. Somatic activities promote a change in focus from weight loss to improved general well-being and bodily functionality. This adjustment in viewpoint may be quite freeing, relieving the tension and frustration that come with plateaus. Individuals may stay motivated and make progress toward their objectives by appreciating their body's possibilities and concentrating on the good parts of the weight reduction process.

In summary, somatic exercises offer a comprehensive approach to breaking through weight loss plateaus, addressing not only the physical but also the emotional and psychological elements of weight reduction. Somatic practices are excellent ways for breaking out of weight loss ruts by increasing bodily awareness, reducing stress, improving sleep, mindful eating, and refocusing on well-being.

Staying Motivated and Engaged

Maintaining motivation and engagement in a weight reduction journey, particularly when combining somatic workouts, provides a unique set of obstacles. The fundamental nature of somatic exercises, which emphasise internal awareness and the mind-body link, necessitates a level of introspection and patience that may appear at odds with the goal-oriented attitude commonly associated with weight reduction. Participants may struggle to retain their excitement over time since the subtle, gradual changes in body awareness and composition may not deliver the same immediate pleasure as more typical, high-intensity workouts. If this disparity is not handled with awareness and strategic ways, it can lead to decreased motivation.

One way is to create realistic and meaningful objectives that go beyond just losing weight. Somatic activities promote a stronger connection with the body, allowing you to recognize and enjoy non-scale successes like better posture, more flexibility, and a higher sense of serenity and well-being. Individuals who appreciate these minor alterations might find satisfaction in the voyage itself, rather than the goal. This shift in viewpoint transforms every somatic session into a chance to discover and connect with the body, maintaining motivation even when weight reduction appears gradual.

Another issue is the seclusion that sometimes comes with somatic practice. Unlike group exercise programmed or team sports, somatic workouts sometimes need a quiet, private environment to concentrate on inward feelings and emotions. This solitude can lower one's morale, especially for people who rely on social support and outward encouragement. Creating a support structure through online networks or finding a physical exercise partner can give the external responsibility and shared experience needed to stay motivated. Sharing successes, obstacles, and insights with others on a similar route may turn the trip into a collaborative experience full of mutual support and understanding.

Variety in somatic practice is also vital for maintaining engagement. While the fundamentals of somatic exercise remain constant, experimenting with new exercises, surroundings, or times of day may keep the practice interesting and dynamic. This may include moving your practice outside on a bright day, attempting somatic exercises in water, or incorporating somatic principles into other sorts of physical activity. Such variation not only reduces boredom, but also enriches the bodily experience by bringing new feelings and challenges, keeping both the mind and body engaged.

The subjective nature of somatic training makes tracking improvement difficult. Traditional weight reduction indicators such as pounds lost or calories burnt may underestimate the benefits of somatic therapies. To address this, people might keep a diary in which they record their experiences, feelings, and observations before and after exercises. Noting changes in emotional well-being, stress levels, bodily awareness, and movement quality gives tangible proof of success, reaffirming the practice's worth and fueling future drive.

Furthermore, the soft nature of somatic workouts may cause people to question their usefulness in weight reduction, thereby reducing desire. Educating oneself on the research underlying somatic techniques can assist. Understanding how these activities lower stress, enhance metabolic function, and foster a more aware connection with food can help legitimize the approach. This information, along with patience and trust in the process, reassures people that they're on the right track for overall health and long-term weight loss.

Finally, combining somatic practices with other weight reduction treatments might help keep motivation high by giving a comprehensive approach to health. Combining somatic exercises with dietary guidance, hydration, sleep, and other types of physical activity results in a total lifestyle transformation that maintains high interest. This holistic approach assures that weight reduction and fitness are more than just about the body; they also involve cultivating the mind and soul. Individuals who face and overcome these problems with smart solutions can stay motivated and involved in their somatic workout journey, resulting in long-term development and a greater respect for their bodies and themselves.

Conclusion

The process of losing weight using somatic workouts implies a significant shift in how people interact with their bodies and approach fitness. This method, which emphasizes mindfulness, bodily awareness, and interior experience, provides a unique approach to weight loss that differs from standard high-intensity workouts. It promotes a delicate yet strong exploration of movement that respects the body's boundaries and recognizes its cues. This method not only helps people lose weight, but it also builds a stronger connection between mind and body, resulting in long-term changes in how they perceive and live in their bodies.

Somatic exercises enable practitioners to shift their focus away from external incentives and goals and towards a deeper knowledge of health and well-being. This shift in attitude is crucial since it emphasizes sustainable approaches over fast cures. The advantages of such activities go beyond the physical, affecting mental and emotional health by lowering stress, boosting mood, and increasing self-esteem. These holistic advantages are critical for everyone on a weight reduction journey since they address the underlying issues that frequently stymie success, such as stress eating and sedentary behavior.

Furthermore, somatic workouts change the way we think about weight reduction progress. It emphasizes that progress is evaluated not just by the scale, but also by a greater awareness of one's physical demands and the capacity to respond to them sensibly. This knowledge leads to improved eating habits, more regular and pleasant physical exercise, and overall greater health. Such findings demonstrate the efficacy of somatic exercises not just as a weight reduction technique, but also as a catalyst for overall lifestyle change.

Somatic exercises' adaptation to individual demands and situations adds to its efficacy as part of a weight loss programmed. Somatic exercises may be modified to match the needs of anybody, from beginners to expert fitness levels, providing a personalized approach that respects the body's existing condition and capacity for growth. This customisation guarantees that the workouts stay accessible and pleasant, which is critical for long-term motivation and adherence.

Somatic workouts also help to develop patience and self-compassion, all of which are necessary for a successful weight reduction journey. Individuals learn to appreciate their bodies and the work they make by concentrating on the present moment and appreciating even minor accomplishments. This good relationship with oneself and one's body can dramatically lessen the probability of sliding into negative behaviors, such as yo-yo diets or obsessive exercise, which frequently sabotage weight reduction efforts.

Furthermore, somatic workouts allow you to smoothly integrate physical activity into your daily life. As these techniques improve body awareness, people naturally choose to move more during the day, whether by stretching, walking, or participating in activities they like. This natural need to move leads to greater physical activity without the need for scheduled training programmed, resulting in weight reduction and enhanced health in a more organic and less forced manner.

To summaries, somatic workouts for weight reduction provide a holistic strategy that extends beyond calorie burning to include mental, emotional, and physical well-being. This programmed teaches important life skills like mindfulness, body awareness, and self-care, which not only aid in weight reduction but also improve overall quality of life. As people continue to practice and incorporate these ideas into their daily lives, they see that somatic exercises are more than simply a means to an end; they are a way to live more completely, healthily, and joyfully. This comprehensive, thoughtful approach to weight reduction and health is a long-term, fulfilling way to achieve and maintain fitness objectives.

15 Days Somatic Workout Tracker

DAILY WORKOUT PLAN

DATE

DAILY MOTIVATION

TODAY'S GOALS

WEATHER

EXECERCISE TYPE

AMOUNT OF WATER

TOTAL :

JOGGING

TOTAL MINUTES

TOTAL STEPS

TODAY'S WORKOUT PLAN

TIME	WORKOUT TYPE

WORKOUT TO GET DONE TODAY

EXERCISE COMPLETED

HEALTHY DIET TRACKER

BREAKFAST	LUNCH
DINNER	SNACKS

NOTES

WORKOUT FOR TOMORROW

DAILY WORKOUT PLAN

DATE

DAILY MOTIVATION

TODAY'S GOALS

WEATHER

EXECERCISE TYPE

AMOUNT OF WATER

TOTAL :

JOGGING

TOTAL MINUTES

TOTAL STEPS

TODAY'S WORKOUT PLAN

TIME	WORKOUT TYPE

WORKOUT TO GET DONE TODAY

EXERCISE COMPLETED

HEALTHY DIET TRACKER

BREAKFAST	LUNCH
DINNER	SNACKS

NOTES

WORKOUT FOR TOMORROW

DAILY WORKOUT PLAN

DATE

DAILY MOTIVATION

WEATHER

TODAY'S GOALS

EXECERCISE TYPE

AMOUNT OF WATER

TOTAL :

JOGGING

TOTAL MINUTES

TOTAL STEPS

TODAY'S WORKOUT PLAN

TIME	WORKOUT TYPE

WORKOUT TO GET DONE TODAY

EXERCISE COMPLETED

HEALTHY DIET TRACKER

BREAKFAST	LUNCH
DINNER	SNACKS

NOTES

WORKOUT FOR TOMORROW

DAILY WORKOUT PLAN

DATE

DAILY MOTIVATION

TODAY'S GOALS

WEATHER

EXECERCISE TYPE

AMOUNT OF WATER

TOTAL :

JOGGING

TOTAL MINUTES

TOTAL STEPS

TODAY'S WORKOUT PLAN

TIME	WORKOUT TYPE

WORKOUT TO GET DONE TODAY

EXERCISE COMPLETED

HEALTHY DIET TRACKER

BREAKFAST	LUNCH
DINNER	SNACKS

NOTES

WORKOUT FOR TOMORROW

DAILY WORKOUT PLAN

DATE

DAILY MOTIVATION

TODAY'S GOALS

WEATHER

EXECERCISE TYPE

AMOUNT OF WATER

TOTAL :

JOGGING

TOTAL MINUTES

TOTAL STEPS

TODAY'S WORKOUT PLAN

TIME	WORKOUT TYPE

WORKOUT TO GET DONE TODAY

EXERCISE COMPLETED

HEALTHY DIET TRACKER

BREAKFAST	LUNCH
DINNER	SNACKS

NOTES

WORKOUT FOR TOMORROW

DAILY WORKOUT PLAN

DATE

DAILY MOTIVATION

TODAY'S GOALS

WEATHER

EXECERCISE TYPE

AMOUNT OF WATER

TOTAL :

JOGGING

TOTAL MINUTES

TOTAL STEPS

TODAY'S WORKOUT PLAN

TIME	WORKOUT TYPE

WORKOUT TO GET DONE TODAY

EXERCISE COMPLETED

HEALTHY DIET TRACKER

BREAKFAST	LUNCH
DINNER	SNACKS

NOTES

WORKOUT FOR TOMORROW

DAILY WORKOUT PLAN

DATE

DAILY MOTIVATION

TODAY'S GOALS

WEATHER

EXECERCISE TYPE

AMOUNT OF WATER

TOTAL :

JOGGING

TOTAL MINUTES

TOTAL STEPS

TODAY'S WORKOUT PLAN

TIME	WORKOUT TYPE

WORKOUT TO GET DONE TODAY

EXERCISE COMPLETED

HEALTHY DIET TRACKER

BREAKFAST	LUNCH
DINNER	SNACKS

NOTES

WORKOUT FOR TOMORROW

DAILY WORKOUT PLAN

DATE

DAILY MOTIVATION

TODAY'S GOALS

WEATHER

EXECERCISE TYPE

AMOUNT OF WATER

TOTAL :

JOGGING

TOTAL MINUTES

TOTAL STEPS

TODAY'S WORKOUT PLAN

TIME	WORKOUT TYPE

WORKOUT TO GET DONE TODAY

EXERCISE COMPLETED

HEALTHY DIET TRACKER

BREAKFAST	LUNCH
DINNER	SNACKS

NOTES

WORKOUT FOR TOMORROW

DAILY WORKOUT PLAN

DATE

DAILY MOTIVATION

TODAY'S GOALS

WEATHER

EXECERCISE TYPE

AMOUNT OF WATER

TOTAL :

JOGGING

TOTAL MINUTES

TOTAL STEPS

TODAY'S WORKOUT PLAN

TIME	WORKOUT TYPE

WORKOUT TO GET DONE TODAY

EXERCISE COMPLETED

HEALTHY DIET TRACKER

BREAKFAST	LUNCH
DINNER	SNACKS

NOTES

WORKOUT FOR TOMORROW

DAILY WORKOUT PLAN

DATE

DAILY MOTIVATION

WEATHER

TODAY'S GOALS

EXECERCISE TYPE

AMOUNT OF WATER

TOTAL :

JOGGING

TOTAL MINUTES

TOTAL STEPS

TODAY'S WORKOUT PLAN

TIME	WORKOUT TYPE

WORKOUT TO GET DONE TODAY

EXERCISE COMPLETED

HEALTHY DIET TRACKER

BREAKFAST	LUNCH
DINNER	SNACKS

NOTES

WORKOUT FOR TOMORROW

DAILY WORKOUT PLAN

DATE

DAILY MOTIVATION

TODAY'S GOALS

WEATHER

EXECERCISE TYPE

AMOUNT OF WATER

TOTAL :

JOGGING

TOTAL MINUTES

TOTAL STEPS

TODAY'S WORKOUT PLAN

TIME	WORKOUT TYPE

WORKOUT TO GET DONE TODAY

EXERCISE COMPLETED

HEALTHY DIET TRACKER

BREAKFAST	LUNCH
DINNER	SNACKS

NOTES

WORKOUT FOR TOMORROW

DAILY WORKOUT PLAN

DATE

DAILY MOTIVATION

TODAY'S GOALS

WEATHER

EXECERCISE TYPE

AMOUNT OF WATER

TOTAL :

JOGGING

TOTAL MINUTES

TOTAL STEPS

TODAY'S WORKOUT PLAN

TIME	WORKOUT TYPE

WORKOUT TO GET DONE TODAY

EXERCISE COMPLETED

HEALTHY DIET TRACKER

BREAKFAST	LUNCH
DINNER	SNACKS

NOTES

WORKOUT FOR TOMORROW

DAILY WORKOUT PLAN

DATE

DAILY MOTIVATION

TODAY'S GOALS

WEATHER

EXECERCISE TYPE

AMOUNT OF WATER

TOTAL :

JOGGING

TOTAL MINUTES

TOTAL STEPS

TODAY'S WORKOUT PLAN

TIME	WORKOUT TYPE

WORKOUT TO GET DONE TODAY

EXERCISE COMPLETED

HEALTHY DIET TRACKER

BREAKFAST	LUNCH
DINNER	SNACKS

NOTES

WORKOUT FOR TOMORROW

DAILY WORKOUT PLAN

DATE

DAILY MOTIVATION

TODAY'S GOALS

WEATHER

EXECERCISE TYPE

AMOUNT OF WATER

TOTAL :

JOGGING

TOTAL MINUTES

TOTAL STEPS

TODAY'S WORKOUT PLAN

TIME	WORKOUT TYPE

WORKOUT TO GET DONE TODAY

EXERCISE COMPLETED

HEALTHY DIET TRACKER

BREAKFAST	LUNCH
DINNER	SNACKS

NOTES

WORKOUT FOR TOMORROW

DAILY WORKOUT PLAN

DATE

DAILY MOTIVATION

TODAY'S GOALS

WEATHER

EXECERCISE TYPE

AMOUNT OF WATER

TOTAL :

JOGGING

TOTAL MINUTES

TOTAL STEPS

TODAY'S WORKOUT PLAN

TIME	WORKOUT TYPE

WORKOUT TO GET DONE TODAY

EXERCISE COMPLETED

HEALTHY DIET TRACKER

BREAKFAST	LUNCH
DINNER	SNACKS

NOTES

WORKOUT FOR TOMORROW

A Group Of Writers Who Take Their Precious Time To Create This Workout Book Have Also Provide You With The Audio Version Of The Book For Free To Enjoy At Your Free Time.

Scan the QR Code Provided below to download it: